RENAL DIET COOKBOOK

MANAGE KIDNEY DISEASE AND AVOID DIALYSIS WITH OVER 100 HEALTHY, LOW SODIUM, LOW POTASSIUM & LOW PHOSPHORUS RECIPES. 4 WEEKS MEAL PLAN INCLUDED

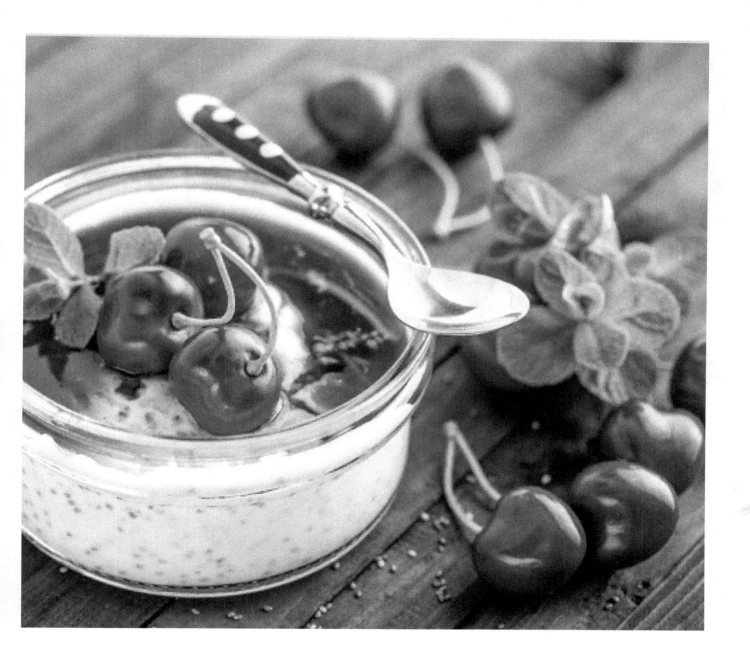

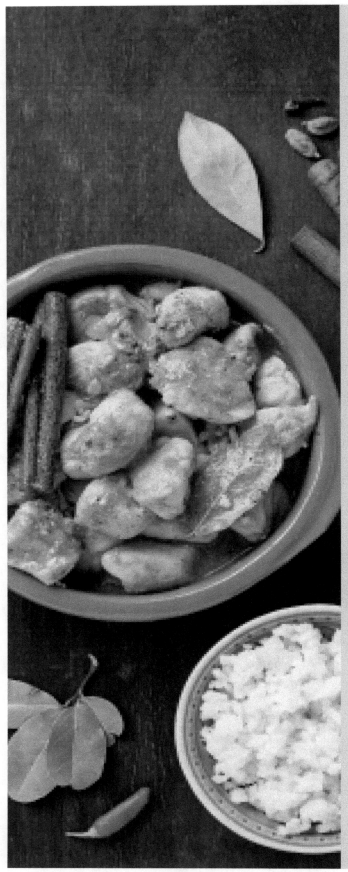

Content

Introduce

If you or someone close to you has been diagnosed with chronic kidney disease (CKD) and are struggling with what to eat, rest assured. You've come to the right place! Nutrition is a powerful weapon in the fight against CKD, and this book has everything you need to harness its power. You might worry that in order to achieve success, you will need to part ways with your favorite foods and commit to a strict and joyless diet forever.

Nutritional counseling provided by a renal expert can help clear up confusion around the renal diet in a couple of sessions. Instead of feeling frustrated and anxious, patients begin to feel confident and motivated in their ability to make the changes necessary for their health. A recent client of mine cried tears of relief at our first appointment because she finally felt confident in her ability to take control of her condition through dietary means. After a few months of following my recommendations, she happily reported improvements in several of her lab values.

A CKD diagnosis can lead to many unwelcome changes in your life, such as frequent doctor visits, needing to take several new medications or the knowledge that your diet needs to be adjusted. With all of this on your plate, it's no wonder that meal preparation can suddenly become a daunting task. This cookbook's purpose is to share with you the wisdom I have gathered from my experience working with patients across the full spectrum of CKD. I'll be keeping the recipes simple, as long lists of ingredients can overwhelm even the most ambitious of cooks. The first recipe you choose is the first step in the right direction. This book will cover the following chapters:

- o Chronic Kidney Disease
- o The Renal Diet
- o Tips for a better Renal Diet
- o Answers to Frequently Asked Questions
- o Weeks Meal plan and Shopping List
- o Breakfast Recipes
- o Smoothies and Drinks Recipes
- o Snacks and sides Recipes
- o Soups and stews Recipes
- o Salads Recipes
- o Vegetables Recipes
- o Meat and Poultry Recipes
- o Desserts Recipes

Chapter 1: Chronic Kidney Disease

There is chronic kidney disease (CKD) when it is damaged kidneys or kidney function decline for three months or more. There are five stages of evolution of a CRM according to the severity of the renal involvement or the degree of deterioration of its function.

Sometimes the kidney failure suddenly occurs. In this case, it is called an acute failure of the kidney. An injury, infection, or something else may be the cause. Acute renal failure is often treated with urgency by dialysis for some time. Often, kidney function recovers itself. Generally, this disease settles slowly and silently, but it progresses over the years. People with CKD do not necessarily go from stage 1 to stage 5 of the disease. Stage 5 of the disease is known under the name of end-stage renal disease (ESRD) or kidney failure in the final stage.

This means that dialysis or the transplanted kidney will "supplement" or "replace" the sick kidneys and do their job.

The Role of the Kidneys in the Body

The Kidneys play a key role in the proper functioning of your body. What most people know is that it helps in filtering out the waste products from the blood and the excess fluid from the blood by flushing it out of the body as urine. What happens is that, as blood is being pumped through the vascular system, it goes through the kidneys to be purified and filtered and then back into the bloodstream.

Aside from that, there are other roles that your kidneys perform like the critical regulation of the body's acid, potassium, and salt content. It also plays a role in the regulation of the production of red blood cells through the production of hormones. It also plays an active role in the promotion of strong and healthy bones by making an active form of vitamin D that helps in controlling the metabolism of calcium—and we all know that calcium is the foundation for a solid bone structure.

The kidneys also play a role in balancing the body's fluids. These help you not to get dehydrated and to support overall body function by having enough fluid in the blood. Further, by regulating the fluid it is also helping to regulate blood pressure, the higher the fluid volume the higher the blood pressure is. The lower the fluid volume the lower your blood pressure is. It also does this through the release of certain hormones that either flushes the water out or reabsorbs the salt minerals and returns it to the vascular system to control fluid volume.

Causes and Risk Factors

What many of us are not aware of is that the cause of kidney disease doesn't necessarily have to occur in the kidneys themselves. Problems affecting our overall health and wellbeing can also induce damage to the kidneys. In the same way, common health problems can also impair the function of these organs. The most frequent causes of kidney disease are hypertension and diabetes.

The pressure from a full bladder can back up and damage or injure kidneys. Let's also not forget the fact that if urine remains in the body for a long time, it can lead to an infection from the fast growth of bacteria and high blood sugar levels. Estimates show that 30% of patients with type 1 diabetes and 10% to 40% of people with type 2 diabetes will eventually experience kidney failure.

Besides diabetes and hypertension, other causes of kidney disease include:

Infection

Renal artery stenosis

Heavy metal poisoning

Lupus

Some drugs

Prolonged obstruction of the urinary tract from conditions such as kidney stones, enlarged prostate, some cancers

Effects and symptoms

Signs and symptoms of kidney disease don't appear suddenly, and they develop over time. Many people don't even know they have kidney disease until it reaches late stages because they are unable to identify some warning signs. Symptoms of kidney diseases may vary from one person to another as well as their severity. But generally speaking, the most common signs of kidney disease include:

Nausea and vomiting

Hypertension that is difficult to control

Loss of appetite

Shortness of breath

Chest pain

Weakness or fatigue

Sleep disturbances

Persistent itching

Changes in how much a patient urinates

Swollen feet and ankles

Reduced mental sharpness

Stages

Chronic kidney disease is categorized into five stages, each one characterized by a certain degree of damage done to the kidneys and rate of glomerular filtration, which is the rate at which filtration takes place in the kidneys. These help us understand just how well the kidneys are functioning.

Stage 1

The first stage is the least severe and actually comes close to a healthy state of your kidneys. Most people will never be aware if they have entered stage 1 of chronic kidney disease or CKD. In many cases, if people discover stage 1 CKD, then it is because they were being tested for diabetes or high blood pressure. Otherwise, people can find out about stage 1 CKD if they discover protein or blood in the urine, signs of kidney damage in an ultrasound, a computerized tomography (CT) scan, or through magnetic resonance imaging (MRI). If people have a family history of polycystic kidney disease (PKD), then there are chances that they might have CKD as well.

Stage 2

In this stage, there is a mild decrease in the glomerular filtration rate. People don't usually notice any symptoms at this stage as well. The reasons for discovering any signs of CKD is the same as with the reasons provided in stage 1.

In stage 1, the glomerular filtration rate (GFR) is around 90 ml/min. The normal range of the GFR is from 90 ml/min to 120 ml/min. So, as you can see, stage 1 CKD shows a GFR at the lower end of the range. Because it falls so close to a normal rate, it easily goes unnoticed. At stage 2, the GFR falls to between 60-89 ml/min. You might become concerned with the range stage 2 falls in, but your kidneys are actually resilient. Even if they are not functioning at 100 percent, your kidneys are capable of doing a good job. So good that you might not notice anything was out of the ordinary.

Stage 3

At this stage, the kidneys suffer moderate damage. In order to properly gauge the level of damage, this stage is further divided into two: stage 3A and stage 3B. The reason for the division is that even though the severity of the disease worsens from 3A to 3B, the damage to the kidneys is still within moderate levels.

Each of the divisions is characterized by their GFR.

3A has a GFR between 45-59 ml/min

3B has a GFR between 30-44 ml/min

When patients reach stage 3, they begin to experience other symptoms of CKD, which include the below:

Increase in fatigue

Shortness of breath and swelling of extremities, also called edema

Slight kidney pain, where the pain is felt in the lower back area

Change in the color of urine

Stage 4
At stage 4, the kidney disease becomes severe. The GFR falls to 15-30 ml/min. As the waste buildup increases. The patient might experience nausea and vomiting, a buildup of urea in the blood that could cause bad breath, and find themselves having trouble doing everyday tasks such as reading a newspaper or trying to write up an email.

It is important to see a nephrologist (a doctor who specializes in kidney problems) when the patient reaches stage 4.

Stage 5
At stage 5, the kidneys have a GFR of less than 15 ml/min. This is a truly low rate that causes the waste buildup to reach a critical point. The organs have reached an advanced stage CKD, causing them to lose almost all their abilities to function normally.

Chapter 2: The Renal Diet

Foods to eat
Cauliflower - 1 cup contains 19 mg sodium, 176 potassium, 40 mg phosphorus

One of the most effective ways to prevent kidney disease is with a proper diet.

It's also important to know that those who are at risk of this disease or have already been diagnosed with this condition can help alleviate symptoms and slow down the progression of the disease with a diet called the renal diet.

A renal diet is a type of diet that involves the consumption of foods and drinks that are low in potassium, sodium, and phosphorus.

It also puts focus on the consumption of high-quality protein as well as limiting too much intake of fluids and calcium.

Since each person's body is different, it's important to come up with a specific diet formulated by a dietician to make sure that the diet is tailored to the needs of the patient.

Some of the substances that you have to check and monitor for proper renal diet include:

The Benefits of Renal Diet
A renal diet minimizes intake of sodium, potassium and phosphorus.

Excessive sodium is harmful to people who have been diagnosed with kidney disease as this causes fluid buildup, making it hard for the kidneys to eliminate sodium and fluid.

Improper functioning of the kidneys can also mean difficulty in removing excess potassium.

When there is too much potassium in the body, this can lead to a condition called hyperkalemia, which can also cause problems with the heart and blood vessels.

Kidneys that are not working efficiently find it difficult to remove excess phosphorus.

High levels of phosphorus excrete calcium from the bones causing them to weaken. This also causes the elevation of calcium deposits in the eyes, heart, lungs, and blood vessels.

Fruit punch

Blueberries - 1 cup contains 1.5 mg sodium, 114 potassium, 18 mg phosphorus

Sea Bass - 3 ounces contain 74 mg sodium, 279 potassium, 211 mg phosphorus

Grapes - 1/2 cup contains 1.5 mg sodium, 144 potassium, 15 mg phosphorus

Egg Whites - 2 egg whites contain 110 mg sodium, 108 potassium, 10 mg phosphorus

Garlic - 3 cloves contain 1.5 mg sodium, 36 potassium, 14 mg phosphorus

Buckwheat - 1/2 cup contains 3.5 mg sodium, 74 potassium, 59 mg phosphorus

Olive Oil - 1 ounce 0.6 mg sodium, 0.3 potassium, 0 mg phosphorus

Bulgur - 1/2 cup contains 4.5 mg sodium, 62 potassium, 36 mg phosphorus

Cabbage - 1 cup contains 13 mg sodium, 119 potassium, 18 mg phosphorus

Skinless chicken - 3 ounces contain 63 mg sodium, 216 potassium, 192 mg phosphorus

Bell peppers - 1 piece contains 3 mg sodium, 156 potassium, 19 mg phosphorus

Onion - 1 piece contains 3 mg sodium, 102 potassium, 20 mg phosphorus

Pineapple - 1 cup contains 2 mg sodium, 180 potassium, 13 mg phosphorus

Cranberries – 1 cup contains 2 mg sodium, 85 potassium, 13 mg phosphorus

Mushrooms – 1 cup contains 6 mg sodium, 170 potassium, 42 mg phosphorus

Foods to Avoid

These foods are known to have high levels of potassium, sodium, or phosphorus:

Soda – Soda is believed to contain up to 100 mg of additive phosphorus per 200 ml.

Avocados - 1 cup contains up to 727 mg of potassium.

Canned foods – Canned foods contain high amounts of sodium so make sure that you avoid using these, or at least, opt for low-sodium versions.

Whole wheat bread – 1 ounce of bread contains 57 mg phosphorus and 69 mg potassium, which is higher compared to white bread.

Brown rice – 1 cup of brown rice contains 154 mg potassium while 1 cup of white rice only has 54 mg potassium.

Bananas – 1 banana contains 422 mg of potassium.

Dairy – Dairy products are high in potassium, phosphorus, and calcium. You can still consume dairy products but you have to limit it. Use dairy milk alternatives like almond milk and coconut milk.

Processed Meats – Processed meats are not advisable for people with kidney problems because of their high content of additives and preservatives.

Pickled and cured foods – These are made using large amounts of salt.

Tomatoes – 1 cup tomato sauce contains up to 900 mg potassium.

Instant meals – Instant meals are known for extremely high amounts of sodium.

Spinach – Spinach contains up to 290 mg potassium per cup. Cooking helps reduce the amount of potassium.

List of Juice and Beverages for the Renal Diet

7 Up

Coffee

Cream Soda

Grape soda

Lemon-Lime soda

Lemonade

Apple juice

Apple sauce

Cranberry juice

Cranberry sauce

Grapefruit juice

Tips to avoid Dialysis through the kidney
Make sure to exercise on a daily basis

Try to avoid smoking altogether

Keep your diabetes in check

Keep your blood pressure in check

Try not to overeat and keep your weight in check

Always try to avoid adding more salt to your diet

Try to avoid excess sugar

Try to be socially active as it will help to lighten your mood

And above all, do the things that you love and try to stay positive all the time.

How to understand the nutrients
Diet will allow you to maintain a good nutritional status and avoid the accumulation of toxic substances that the kidney is not able to eliminate.

Rice, pasta, bread, and cereals
They can be consumed once a day, and constitute a good source of energy, especially for those who should limit protein intake; although if the patient is overweight or diabetes should consult the doctor about how much he can take. In any case, these foods should not be integral, since the integral products have a high content of phosphorus and potassium.

Meats
The diet of patients with renal insufficiency should be low in protein, so it is convenient to reduce the consumption of meat and fish to 100 grams daily. In particular, it is important to limit the consumption of red meat, as a study by the University of Singapore warned, which stated that the habitual consumption of this type of meat could increase the risk of the end-stage renal disease up to 40%. Poultry can be an alternative to pigs.

Vegetables
They are, along with fruits, the richest foods in potassium, so you should also take precautions in their consumption, such as letting them soak for a minimum of three hours or give one or two boils, changing the water, so that they lose part Potassium If they are canned you should not drink the juice because it contains the potassium that the vegetable has lost cooked to make sauces or soups.

Carbohydrates
Its intake is not limited, unless the patient is diabetic or obese, or presents any other contraindication that will be assessed by the doctor. They must therefore be consumed daily, to provide the body with the necessary energy. Carbohydrates can be fast-acting, such as sweets (sugar, cookies, jam, honey ...), or slow-acting and, therefore, with an easier energy supply, such as pasta, bread, rice or potatoes.

Liquids
When the patient follows a dialysis treatment, he must control the amount of liquids he ingests, including not only water, but other products such as juices, broths and soups, milk, fruit, coffee or tea and, in general, any beverage. This is because the loss of kidney functionality causes fluid retention to occur between one dialysis session and the next, and causes swelling and hypertension.

Salt
Food should be cooked without salt because the body has difficulty removing sodium, and its accumulation can cause fluid retention and edema formation, increasing the workload of the heart, which could lead to heart failure. In substitution of salt, herbs and spices can be used to season foods, such as bay leaves, basil, thyme, pepper, nutmeg, as well as olive oil and vinegar.

Lifestyle to reduce your kidney problems
Learning that you are suffering from kidney failure might be a difficult thing to cope with. No matter how long you

have been preparing for the inevitable, this is something that will come as a shock to you.

Don't Stress During Kidney Failure

When you are suffering from kidney failure, it's normal to be stressed out all the time. This might lead you to skip meals or even forgetting your medication, which might affect your health even more.

Make sure to involve yourself in regular exercise. Take a hike, ride a bicycle, or just simply take a jog. They all help. And if those aren't your thing, then you can always go for something more soothing, like tai chi or yoga.

When you are feeling too stressed, try to call up a friend or a beloved family member and talk to them. And if that's not helping, you can always take help from a psychiatrist/counselor.

Exercise

Apart from the special diet, such as the Renal Diet, physical activity is another way through which you can improve the quality of your life.

In fact, a study has shown that people who try to complete 10,1000 steps per day and work out for about 21/2 hours every week, while cutting down 500-800 calories per day and following a proper diet routine, have a 50% chance of reducing blood sugar to normal levels, which will further help you to stay healthy.

Avoid Anxiety and Depression

These two are possibly the most prominent issues that you are going to face. A feeling of depression might last for a long time if left unattended. Anxiety might come at the same time, but it won't last for long.

Either way, mood swings will occur that will suddenly make you sad.

Regardless, the main thing to know is that you are not alone in this fight. Thousands of people have and are going through the same experience. Many people often feel left alone and lose the will to fight, but it doesn't have to be the same for you.

It doesn't matter what your situation is; if you just reach out to the right person, then you will always find the help and support that you need.

How to manage your kidney diet when you have diabetes.

A kidney disease diagnosis can seem devastating at first. The news may come as a shock for some people, who may not have experienced any symptoms. It's important to remember that you can control your progress and improvement through diet and lifestyle changes, even when a prognosis is serious. Taking steps to improve your health can make a significant effort to slow the progression of kidney disease and improve your quality of life.

Focus on Weight Loss

Losing weight is one of the most common reasons for going on a diet. It's also one of the best ways to treat kidney disease and prevent further damage. Carrying excess weight contributes to high toxicity levels in the body, by storing toxins instead of releasing them through the kidneys. Eating foods high in trans fats, sugar, and excess sodium contribute to obesity, which affects close to one-third of North Americans and continues to rise in many other countries, where fast foods are becoming easier to access and less expensive. Losing weight is a difficult cycle for many, who often diet temporarily only to return to unhealthy habits after reaching a milestone, which results in gaining the weight back, thus causing an unhealthy "yo-yo" diet effect.

Quit Smoking and Reduce Alcohol

It's not easy to quit smoking or using recreational drugs, especially where there has been long-term use and the effects have already made an impact on your health. At some point, you'll begin to notice a difference in the way you feel and how your body changes over time. This includes chronic coughing related to respiratory conditions, shortness of breath, and a lack of energy. These changes may be subtle at first, and it may appear as though there is minimal damage or none at all, though smoking inevitably catches up with age and contributes to the development of cancer, premature aging, and kidney damage. The more toxins we consume or add to our body, the more challenging it becomes for the kidneys to work efficiently, which eventually slows their ability to function.

Track your progress on a calendar or in a notebook, either by pen and paper or on an application. This can serve as a motivator, as well as a means to display how you've done so far and where you can improve. For example, you may have reduced your smoking from ten to seven cigarettes per day, then increased to nine.

This may indicate a slight change that can keep in mind to focus on reducing your intake further, from nine cigarettes to seven or six per day, and so on.

Don't be afraid to ask for help. Many people cannot quit on their own without at least some assistance from others. Seeking the guidance and expertise of a counselor or medical professional to better yourself can be one of the most important decisions you make to improve the quality of your life.

Sodium

Sodium is an important mineral that helps regulate your body's water content and blood pressure. Sodium is also a major electrolyte, which helps control the fluid in the body's tissues and cells. When your kidneys are working the way they are supposed to, they can remove sodium from the body as needed. However, much like phosphorus, when your kidneys are not working properly the sodium build up in your body and make your blood pressure rise, make you thirsty, and result in water retention, causing you to gain weight.

For people in the early stages of chronic kidney disease—stages 1, 2, or 3— it is suggested that you restrict your sodium intake to between 2,000 mg and 3,000 mg per day. If you have stage 4 or 5 chronic kidney disease and require dialysis, even lower amounts may be prescribed. It is recommended that you consume no more than 1,500 mg of sodium per day.

Potassium

Potassium is an important mineral that participates in many functions, including muscle function, and it helps promote a healthy heartbeat. Like sodium, potassium is also necessary for fluid and electrolyte balance.

While potassium is needed for our health, patients with kidney disease do need to reduce the intake of this mineral. The reason is simple; when kidneys are damaged, they are not able to eliminate excess potassium out of the body. This causes a buildup of potassium and leads to other problems such as muscle weakness, heart attack, slow pulse, irregular heartbeat.

Chapter 3: Tips for a better Renal Diet

Apart from regulating fluids in the body, it also aids the body in passing messages between the body and the brain. Just like sodium, potassium is classified as an electrolyte, a term used to refer to a family of minerals that react in water. When potassium is dissolved in water, it produces positively charged ions. Using these ions, potassium can conduct electricity, which allows it to carry out some incredibly important functions. Take for example the messages that are communicated between the brain and the body. These messages are sent back and forth in the form of impulses. But one has to wonder; what exactly creates those impulses? It's not like our body has an inbuilt electrical generator.

Phosphorus

Phosphorus is a mineral required for the maintenance and development of bones. This mineral also participates in the development of connective tissues, takes part in muscle movement, and so much more. Damaged kidneys don't remove excess phosphorus from the body. In turn, levels of this mineral accumulate and impair calcium balance, thus causing weak bones and calcium deposits in blood vessels.

This mineral makes up about 1% of your body weight. That may not seem like a lot in actuality, but remember that our body consists of a lot of water. For this reason, oxygen makes up 62% of our total body weight, followed by carbon at 18%, hydrogen at 9%, and nitrogen at 3%. But guess which are the next two major elements in the human body?

Calcium at 1.5%.

Phosphorus at 1%.

So, you see, even though phosphorus makes up just 1% of the total body weight, it is still a significant element.

What is it used for?

Let me put it this way. Phosphorus is one of the reasons by you can smile wide. It is the reason your skin and other parts of the body are the way they are and do not just fall on the floor, like the way a piece of cloth might when you drop it. Phosphorus is responsible for the formation of your teeth and the bones that keep your body structure the way it currently is.

When kidney problems strike us, we don't need the extra amount of phosphorus. While phosphorus is truly important for our bones and teeth, an excessive amount in the blood can lead to weaker bones. Since most of the food that we eat already includes phosphorus, we are going to try and avoid anything that has a high percentage of the mineral.

Protein

Protein plays an important role in the body and they are crucial to staying healthy. It allows your body to counter-act everyday wear and tear, heal from injury, stop bleeding, and fight infections. However, too much protein can put a strain on your kidneys, and even cause additional damage. You can talk with your healthcare provider about how a reduced protein diet may help slow the progression of CKD. If you're in the early stages of chronic kidney disease, such as stages 1 and 2, your protein intake will be limited to 12 to 15 percent of your calorie intake each day, which is the same level recommended by the Dietary Reference Intakes (DRIs) for a healthy diet for normal adults. People receiving dialysis should take in about 1.2 grams of protein per kilogram of body weight each day (1 kilogram is about 2.2 pounds). For those in stages 3 and 4, recommended protein intake is between 0.6 and 0.75 g/kg, according to the Kidney Disease Outcomes Quality Initiative (KDOQI) of The National Kidney Foundation.

As you choose your protein sources, it's important to know that some foods contain more useful and healthy proteins than others.

Fluids

Water sustains us. After all, 60% of the human adult's body is composed of water. This is why you might have heard of popular recommendations on how you should be having about eight glasses of water per day.

When you have kidney disease, you may not need as much fluid as you did before. The reason for this is that damaged kidneys do not dispose of extra fluids as well as they should. All the extra fluid in your body could be dangerous. It could cause swelling in various areas, high blood pressure, and heart problems. Fluid can also build up around your lungs, preventing you from breathing normally.

There is no measurement of how much fluid is considered as extra fluid. I strongly suggest that you should visit the doctor and get more information about fluid retention from him or her. The doctor will be able to guide you better and help you understand how many fluids you might require. The thing to understand here is that many of the foods that we eat, including fruits, vegetables, and most soups, have a water content in them as well. Getting to know your kidney's ability to hold on to fluids will aid you in preparing or planning better meals for yourself.

Tips for eating out

Portion control

Portion control is an important part of the RENAL diet because it will help you to understand the serving size of food, the number of calories the food contains, and the energy of food. It is also important for the management of your body weight. Portion control means the balance of calories and a healthy combination of food items. The food pyramid may help you to understand the healthy balance of each food item. The portion control can be disturbed due to some emotional factors, including depressed mood and monotony in food items. The RENAL diet is designed with a combination of your favorite food items; therefore, you will not feel any boredom in the diet.

Chapter 4: Answers to Frequently Asked Questions

What is the maximum potassium daily limit?

When following a renal diet, you ideally want to make sure that potassium levels are below 250mg/per serving or up to 7% of the food's total nutritional value.

Can I lose weight with a renal diet?

The number of calories that you need to take depends on your age, gender, health status, and weight goal. If you want to lose weight on your renal diet plan, then discuss it with a nutritionist.

Does my CKD stage count when following a renal diet?

Yes. In earlier stages (1 to 3), it is fine to consume low to moderate amounts of sodium, potassium, and phosphorus, while your fluid intake should be up to 2.5 liters per day. However, if you are in dialysis, then you have to limit all the above minerals.

Is it okay to take caffeine in a renal diet?

During the first three stages of CKD, a caffeine-based drink is perfectly fine. You may drink up to 2 cups of coffee per day without any worries.

How about over the counter medication?

Counter medication/painkillers like aspirin and ibuprofen are not indicated for CKD patients. Any drug that belongs in the nonsteroidal anti-inflammatory drugs category should be avoided.

Are Sodas Bad for a Kidney?

When considering sodas, make sure that you avoid dark sodas, such as Pepsi or Coca Cola as they include phosphorus additives that are extremely harmful to your kidneys. Replace them with Cherry 7 Up, 7 Up, cream soda, ginger ale, sprite, etc. But even so, make sure to have them in very small amounts, as little as possible.

Is Cheese Allowed or Completely Forbidden?

As a rule of thumb, cheese should be avoided as it contains large amounts of phosphorus. However, some cheese is lower in phosphorus, such as cream cheese, Swiss Cheese, Natural Cheese, etc. One or two ounces of those once in a while won't hurt you.

What Are Some of the Precautions That I Can Take?

There are multiple steps that you can take to protect your kidneys. Some include:

Follow a kidney-friendly diet, such as the renal diet

Make sure to keep your blood pressure under control

Stop smoking

Keep your blood glucose level under check

Is There A Permanent Cure for CKD?

Unfortunately, no. Just like Asthma, once you get affected by CKD, you can only hope to keep it under check through proper management. There is no known permanent treatment at the moment.

What Are the Most Common Medications That I Should Avoid?

Some common medications to avoid that might lead to kidney diseases include:

Over the counter painkillers

Laxatives

Enemas

Anti-Inflammatory medicines

Food supplements

Chapter 5: 4 Weeks Meal plan and Shopping List

Vitamin and herbal medications

Always make sure to consult your Nephrologist before taking any over the counter medicine that might fall into any of the above categories.

What Are Some Common Tests to Assess Kidney Functions?

Some common tests to check the condition of your kidney include:

Blood tests that specifically look for BUN, Electrolytes, and Serum Creatinine.

Urine tests that check for Glomerular Filtration rate and Microalbumin.

Imaging tests such as renal ultrasound, CT Scan, or MRI.

Kidney biopsy, where a small part of your kidney is removed by a needle to know if it is affected.

DAY	BREAKFAST	LUNCH/DINNER	DESSERT
1	Egg Cups	Authentic Shrimp Wraps	Authentic Shrimp Wraps
2	Breakfast Casserole	Loveable Tortillas	Loveable Tortillas
3	Grilled Veggie and Cheese Bagel	Elegant Veggie Tortillas	Elegant Veggie Tortillas
4	Cauliflower Tortilla	Delightful Pizza	Delightful Pizza
5	Eggs Benedict	Winner Kabobs	Winner Kabobs
6	Cranberry and Apple Oatmeal	Tempting Burgers	Tempting Burgers
7	Blueberry Breakfast Smoothie	Tastiest Meatballs	Tastiest Meatballs
8	Waffles	Salad with Strawberries and Goat Cheese	Salad with Strawberries and Goat Cheese
9	Apple Sauce Cream Toast	Pork Chops and Apples	Pork Chops and Apples
10	Mini Frittatas	Pan Fried Beef and Broccoli	Pan Fried Beef and Broccoli
11	Egg Whites and Veggie Bake	Ground Turkey Burger	Ground Turkey Burger
12	Zucchini Bake	One Portion Frittatas	One Portion Frittatas

13	Hot Cereal Meal	Ground Beef Soup	Ground Beef Soup
14	Peach Pancakes	Salmon with Spicy Honey	Salmon with Spicy Honey
15	Crispy Veggie Bake	Stuffed Peppers	Stuffed Peppers
16	Strawberry Cream French Toast	Rigatoni Spring Pasta	Rigatoni Spring Pasta
17	Spaghetti Frittata	Zucchini and Carrots Rosemary Chicken	Zucchini and Carrots Rosemary Chicken
19	Veggie Mushroom Omelet	Turkey Sausages	Turkey Sausages
21	Mini Frittatas	Braised Cabbage	Braised Cabbage
22	Egg Whites and Veggie Bake	Simple Broccoli Stir-Fry	Simple Broccoli Stir-Fry
23	Egg Cups	Tangy Mushroom Stir-Fry	Tangy Mushroom Stir-Fry
24	Breakfast Casserole	Perfect Zucchini Stir-Fry	Perfect Zucchini Stir-Fry
25	Grilled Veggie and Cheese Bagel	Authentic Shrimp Wraps	Authentic Shrimp Wraps
26	Cauliflower Tortilla	Loveable Tortillas	Loveable Tortillas
27	Eggs Benedict	Elegant Veggie Tortillas	Elegant Veggie Tortillas
	Cranberry and Apple Oatmeal	Delightful Pizza	Delightful Pizza
28	Blueberry Breakfast Smoothie	Winner Kabobs	Winner Kabobs
29	Waffles	Tempting Burgers	Tempting Burgers
	Apple Sauce Cream Toast	Tastiest Meatballs	Tastiest Meatballs
30	Mini Frittatas	Salad with Strawberries and Goat Cheese	Salad with Strawberries and Goat Cheese

Shopping list

The renal diet contains fresh fruits, vegetables, whole-grain items, and lots of other healthy options. You can make your shopping faster and easier by preparing a list of a diet food items. While shopping grocery items for your diet, you have to consider the following tips:

Plan your regular meals according to the fresh foods and vegetables of the season.

Whole-grain foods, such as whole-wheat pasta, bread, brown rice, quinoa, and barely should be an important part of your meal.

To prepare a delicious and filling meal, you can use beans, peas and lentils full of protein and fiber.

Buy fresh lean meats, poultry without skin, seafood, and tofu.

Buy low-fat and fat-free dairy food items for regular servings.

Low-sodium canned tomatoes, sauce, vegetables, beans, soups, and broth can be bought for your meals.

Low-calorie beverages, such as low-fat and fat-free milk should be part of your shopping. Try to get fresh fruit juice, low-sodium, vegetable juices, herbal tea, and mineral water.

You can also buy low-fat dressings and containments.

Chapter 6:
Breakfast Recipes

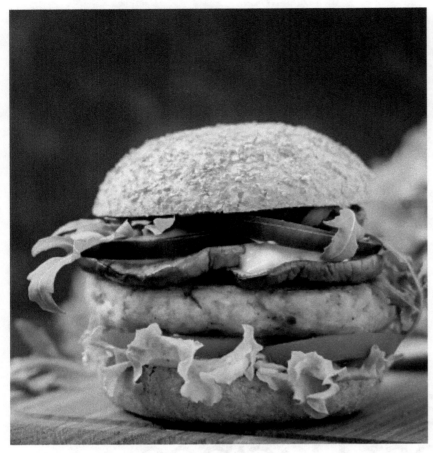

INGREDIENTS

o 1 eggplant, trimmed

o 10 oz of chicken fillet

o 1 teaspoon of Plain yogurt

o 1/2 teaspoon of minced garlic

o 1 tablespoon of fresh cilantro, chopped

o 2 lettuce leaves

o 1 teaspoon of olive oil

o 1/2 teaspoon of salt

o 1/2 teaspoon of chili pepper

o 1 teaspoon of butter

DIRECTIONS

1. Slice the eggplant lengthwise into 4 slices.

2. Rub the eggplant slices with minced garlic and brush with olive oil.

3. Grill the eggplant slices on the preheated to 375F grill for 3 minutes from each side.

4. Meanwhile, rub the chicken fillet with salt and chili pepper.

5. Place it in the skillet and add butter.

6. Roast the chicken for 6 minutes from each side over the medium-high heat.

7. Cool the cooked eggplants gently and spread one side of them with Plain yogurt.

8. Add lettuce leaves and chopped fresh cilantro.

9. After this, slice the cooked chicken fillet and add over the lettuce.

10. Cover it with the remaining sliced eggplant to get the sandwich shape. Pin the sandwich with the toothpick if needed.

Eggplant Chicken Sandwich

PREPARATION
10 MIN

COOKING
15 MIN

SERVES FOR
2 PEOPLE

NUTRITION: calories 368, fat 15.2, fiber 8.2, carbs 14.2, protein 43.5

Strawberry Muesli

INGREDIENTS

- 2 cups of Greek yogurt
- 1 1/2 cup of strawberries, sliced
- 1 1/2 cup of Muesli
- 4 teaspoon of maple syrup
- 3/4 teaspoon of ground cinnamon

DIRECTIONS

1. Put Greek yogurt in the food processor.
2. Add 1 cup of strawberries, maple syrup, and ground cinnamon.
3. Blend the ingredients until you get smooth mass.
4. Transfer the yogurt mass in the serving bowls.
5. Add Muesli and stir well.
6. Leave the meal for 30 minutes in the fridge.
7. After this, decorate it with the remaining sliced strawberries.

PREPARATION
10 MIN

COOKING
30 MIN

SERVES FOR
4 PEOPLE

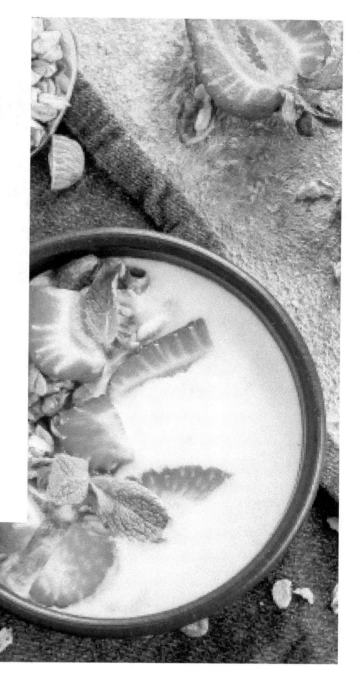

NUTRITION: calories 149, fat 2.6, fiber 3.6, carbs 21.6, protein 12

Yogurt Bulgur

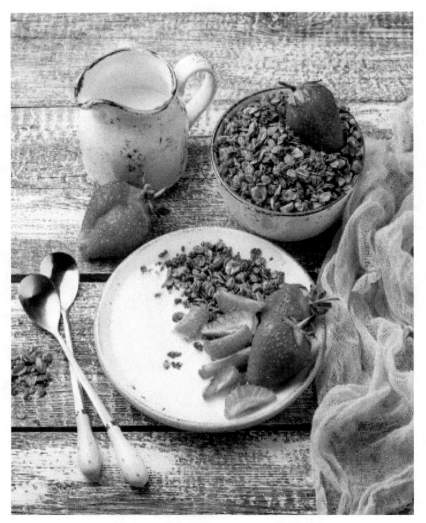

INGREDIENTS

o   1 cup of bulgur

o   2 cups of Greek yogurt

o   1 1/2 cup of water

o   1/2 teaspoon of salt

o   1 teaspoon of olive oil

DIRECTIONS

1.   Pour olive oil into the saucepan and add bulgur.

2.   Roast it over medium heat for 2-3 minutes. Stir it from time to time.

3.   After this, add salt and water.

4.   Close the lid and cook bulgur for 15 minutes over medium heat.

5.   Then chill the cooked bulgur well and combine it with Greek yogurt. Stir it carefully.

6.   Transfer the cooked meal into the serving plates. The yogurt bulgur tastes the best when it is cold.

NUTRITION: calories 274, fat 4.9, fiber 8.5, carbs 40.8, protein 19.2

PREPARATION
10 MIN

COOKING
15 MIN

SERVES FOR
3 PEOPLE

Chia Pudding

INGREDIENTS

- 1/2 cup of raspberries
- 2 teaspoons of maple syrup
- 1 1/2 cup of Plain yogurt
- 1/4 teaspoon of ground cardamom
- 1/3 cup of Chia seeds, dried

DIRECTIONS:

1. Mix up together Plain yogurt with maple syrup and ground cardamom.

2. Add Chia seeds. Stir it gently.

3. Put the yogurt in the serving glasses and top with the raspberries.

4. Refrigerate the breakfast for at least 30 minutes or overnight.

PREPARATION
10 MIN

COOKING
30 MIN

SERVES FOR
2 PEOPLE

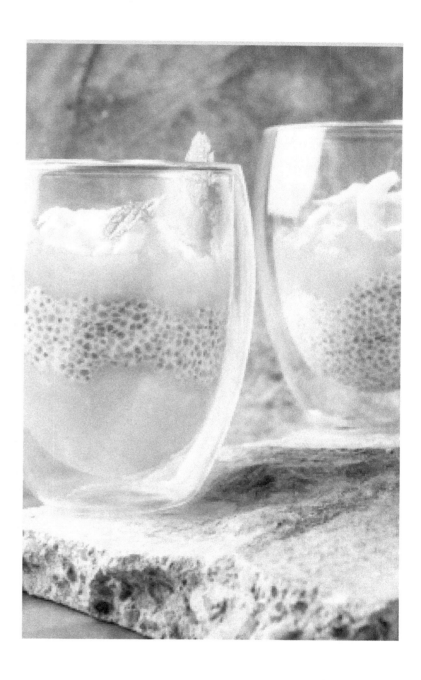

NUTRITION: calories 303, fat 11.2, fiber 11.8, carbs 33.2, protein 15.5

Yufka Pies

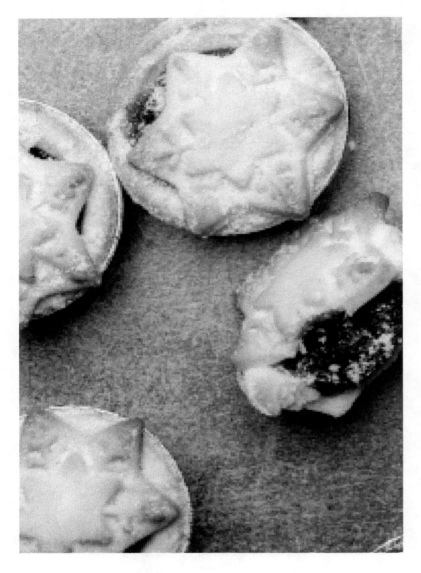

INGREDIENTS

- o 7 oz yufka dough/phyllo dough
- o 1 cup of Cheddar cheese, shredded
- o 1 cup of fresh cilantro, chopped
- o 2 eggs, beaten
- o 1 teaspoon of paprika
- o 1/4 teaspoon of chili flakes
- o 1/2 teaspoon of salt
- o 2 tablespoons of sour cream
- o 1 teaspoon of olive oil

DIRECTIONS

1. In the mixing bowl, combine sour cream, salt, chili flakes, paprika, and beaten eggs.
2. Brush the springform pan with olive oil.
3. Place 1/4 part of all yufka dough in the pan and sprinkle it with 1/4 part of the egg mixture.
4. Add a 1/4 cup of cheese and 1/4 cup of cilantro.
5. Cover the mixture with 1/3 part of the remaining yufka dough and repeat all the steps again. You should get 4 layers.
6. Cut the yufka mixture into 6 pies and bake at 360F for 20 minutes. The cooked pies should have a golden-brown color.

PREPARATION
15 MIN

COOKING
20 MIN

SERVES FOR
6 PEOPLE

NUTRITION: calories 213, fat 11.4, fiber 0.8, carbs 18.2, protein 9.1

Breakfast Potato Latkes with Spinach

INGREDIENTS

o 2 potatoes, peeled

o 1/2 onion, diced

o 1/2 cup of spinach, chopped

o 2 eggs, beaten

o 1/2 teaspoon of salt

o 1/2 teaspoon of ground black pepper

o 1 teaspoon of olive oil

DIRECTIONS

1. Grate the potato and mix it with chopped spinach, diced onion, salt, and ground black pepper.

2. Add eggs and stir until homogenous.

3. Then pour olive oil into the skillet and preheat it well.

4. Make the medium latkes with the help of two spoons and transfer them in the preheated oil.

5. Roast the latkes for 3 minutes from each side or until they are golden brown.

6. Dry the cooked latkes with the help of a paper towel if needed.

PREPARATION
10 MIN

COOKING
6 MIN

SERVES FOR
4 PEOPLE

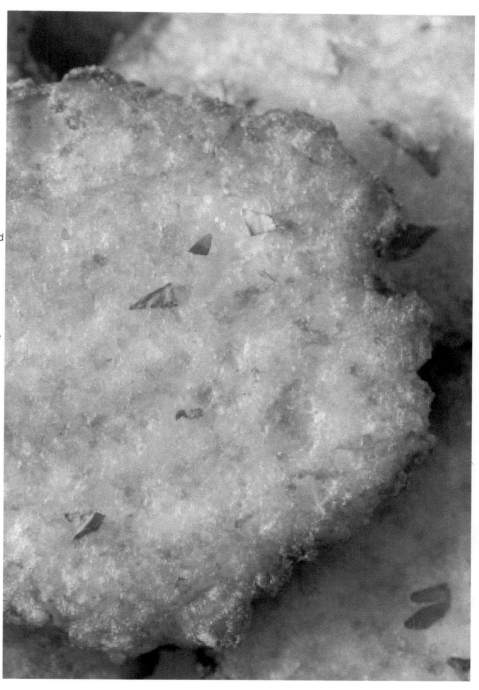

NUTRITION: calories 122, fat 3.5, fiber 3, carbs 18.5, protein 4.9

Egg White Scramble

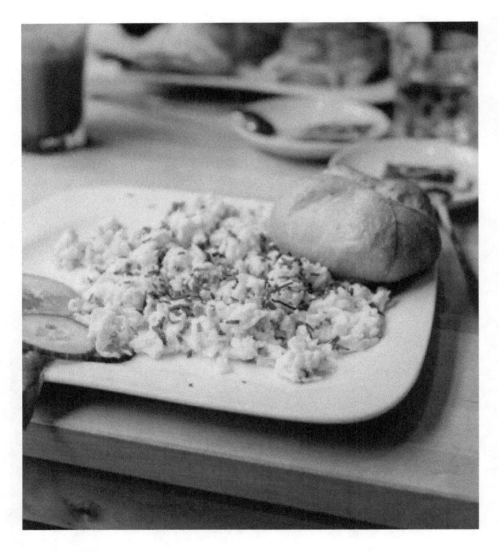

INGREDIENTS

o 1 teaspoon almond butter

o 4 egg whites

o 1/4 teaspoon of salt

o 1/2 teaspoon of paprika

o 2 tablespoons of heavy cream

DIRECTIONS

1. Whisk the egg whites gently and add heavy cream.

2. Put the almond butter in the skillet and melt it.

3. Then add egg white mixture.

4. Sprinkle it with salt and cook for 2 minutes over medium heat.

5. After this, scramble the egg whites with the help of the fork or spatula and sprinkle with paprika.

6. Cook the scrambled egg whites for 3 minutes more.

7. Transfer the meal into the serving plates.

PREPARATION
10 MIN

COOKING
6 HR

SERVES FOR
4 PEOPLE

NUTRITION: calories 68, fat 5.1, fiber 0.5, carbs 1.3, protein 4.6

Chia Bars

INGREDIENTS

- o 11/2 cups of dates, pitted and chopped
- o 1/2 cup of chia seeds
- o 1/3 cup of cocoa powder
- o 1/2 cup of shredded coconut, unsweetened
- o 1 cup of chopped walnuts
- o 1/2 cup of oats
- o 1/2 cup of dark chocolate, chopped
- o 1 teaspoon of vanilla extract

DIRECTIONS

1. In your food processor, mix the dates with the chia seeds, cocoa, coconut, walnuts, oats, chocolate, and vanilla. Pulse well then press into a lined baking dish. Keep in the freezer for 4 hours, cut into 12 bars and serve for breakfast.

2. Enjoy!

PREPARATION
4 HR

COOKING
0 MIN

SERVES FOR
4 PEOPLE

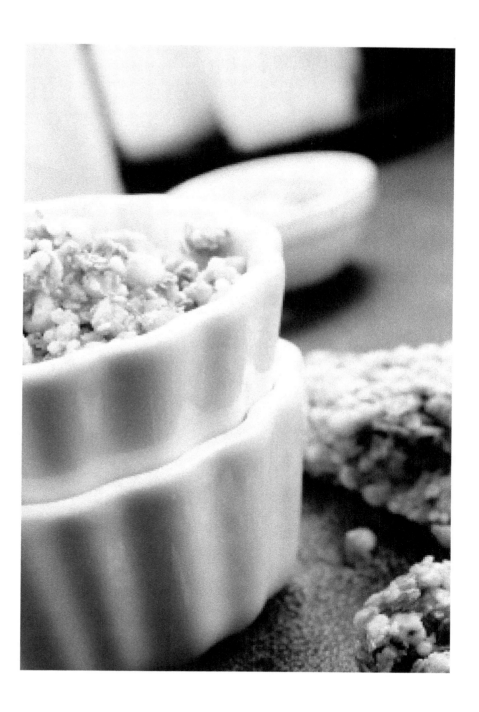

NUTRITION: calories 125, fat 5, fiber 4, carbs 12, protein 5

Shrimp Bok Choy

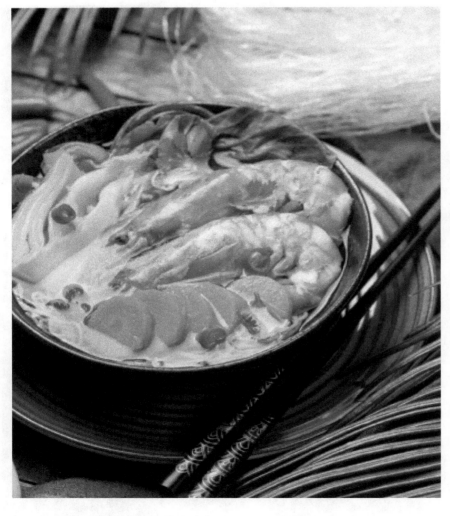

INGREDIENTS

o   2 tablespoons of coconut oil

o   2 crushed garlic cloves

o   1 1/2 inch piece of freshly grated ginger

o   1/2 pound trimmed and thinly sliced Bok Choy

o   1 teaspoon of cayenne pepper

o   1 tablespoon of oyster sauce

o   Ground black pepper and salt to taste

o   10 ounces peeled and deveined shrimp

DIRECTIONS

1. Put a pan on medium heat and warm up the coconut oil. Cook the garlic until it is slightly brown.

2. Mix in the ginger and the Bok Choy. Then put in the cayenne pepper, oyster sauce, pepper, and salt. Stir while cooking for another 5 minutes. Put on a serving plate.

3. Heat the other tablespoon of coconut oil in the pan and cook the shrimp, while stirring every now and then. It should take around 3 minutes for the shrimp to turn pink and opaque.

4. Put the shrimp on top of the Bok Choy and serve with lemon wedges.

PREPARATION
8 MIN

COOKING
15 MIN

SERVES FOR
24 PEOPLE

NUTRITION: Calories 171, Protein 18.9g, Fat 8.4g, Carbs 5.8g

Cauliflower and Mushroom Casserole

INGREDIENTS

- o 2 tablespoons of lard
- o 1 teaspoon of yellow mustard
- o 1 tablespoon of Piri Piri sauce
- o 1 cup of aged goat cheese
- o 1 cup of chicken stock
- o 4 lightly beaten eggs
- o 1/2 Cup of sour cream
- o Cup chive & onion cream cheese
- o 1/2 pound thinly sliced brown Cremini mushrooms
- o 1 teaspoon of fresh or dry rosemary, minced
- o 1/3 teaspoon of freshly ground pepper
- o 1/2 teaspoon of salt
- o 1 large head of cauliflower florets

DIRECTIONS

1. Preheat the oven to 3000F. Spray a casserole dish with nonstick cooking spray.

2. Preheat a pan over medium heat and then melt the lard. Put in the mustard, Piri Piri sauce, goat cheese, cream cheese, sour cream, chicken stock, and eggs. Cook these until they're hot.

3. In the baking dish, layer the cauliflower with the mushrooms. Season with pepper, salt and rosemary.

4. Put the other mixture on top of the vegetables and cook for 25 – 30 minutes. Best served hot.

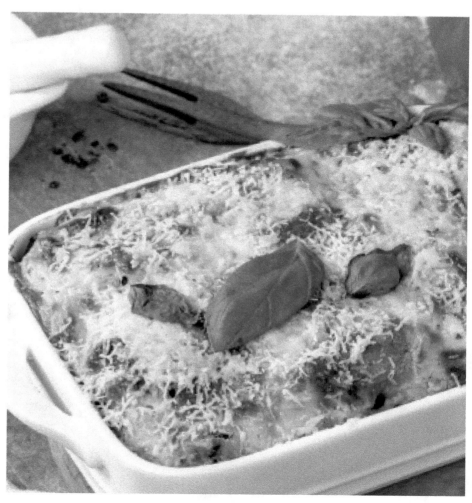

PREPARATION
8 MIN

COOKING
35 MIN

SERVES FOR
2 PEOPLE

NUTRITION: Calories 275, Protein 14g, Fat 21.3g Carbs, 5.3g, Sugar 2.6g

Cheddar and Spinach Muffins

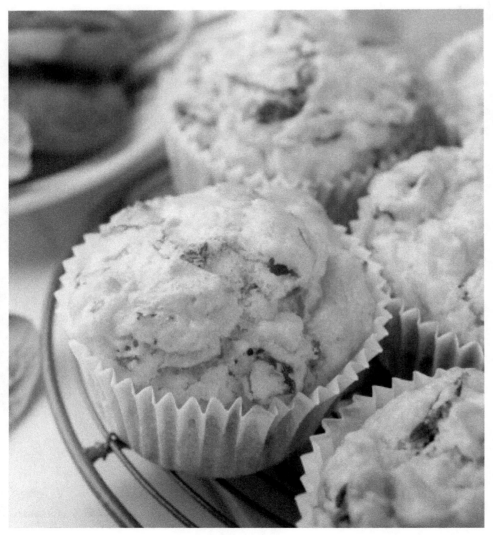

INGREDIENTS

o   8 eggs

o   1 cup of full-fat milk

o   2 tablespoons of olive oil

o   1/4 teaspoon of ground black pepper

o   1/3 teaspoon of salt

o   1 cup chopped spinach

o   1 1/2 cups of grated cheddar cheese

DIRECTIONS

1. Put your oven on to 3500F.

2. Mix together the oil, eggs and milk. Add the pepper and salt, the spinach and the cheese. Combine well.

3. Put the mixture into a greased muffin tin.

4. Put in the oven and bake for 25 minutes. The muffins should spring back when touched.

PREPARATION
8 MIN

COOKING
30 MIN

SERVES FOR
6 PEOPLE

NUTRITION: Calories 252, Protein 16.1g, Fat 19.7g, Carbs 3g, Sugar 1.6g

Muffins with Kale and Gruyère Cheese

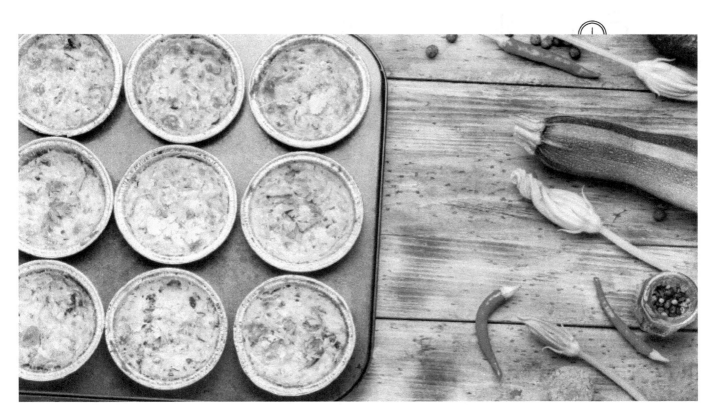

INGREDIENTS

o   1/2 cup of full-fat milk

o   1/2 teaspoon of dried basil

o   1 1/2 cup of grated Gruyere cheese

o   Sea salt to taste

o   5 eggs

o   1/2 pound chopped prosciutto

o   10 ounces cooked and drained kale

DIRECTIONS

1.   Preheat the oven to 3600F. Spray a muffin tin with a nonstick cooking spray.

2.   Whisk together the eggs, milk, basil, Gruyere cheese, and salt. Then put in the prosciutto and the kale. Put the mixture in the muffin tin, making sure that each muffin cup is filled 3/4 full.

3.   Bake for around 25 minutes. They are good served with sour cream.

NUTRITION: Calories 275 Protein 21.6, Fat 15.8g, Carbs 2.2g, Sugar 0.4g

Chapter 7: Smoothies and Drinks Recipes
Peach Smoothie

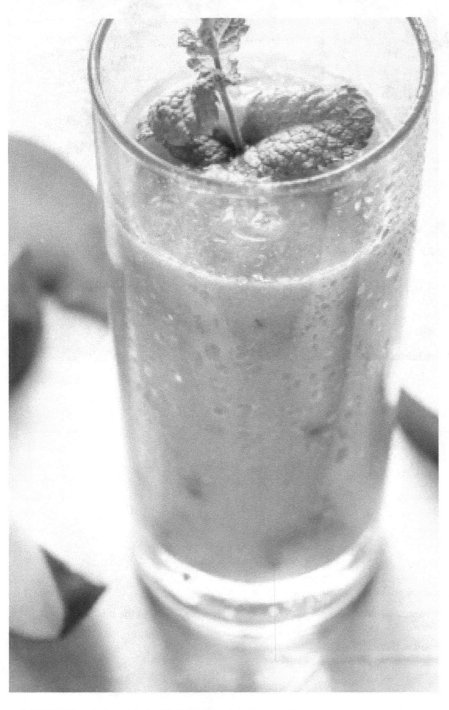

INGREDIENTS

o 3/4 cup fresh peaches, diced

o 1 tablespoon of Splenda granulated sugar

o 2 tablespoons of powdered egg whites

o 1/2 cup of ice

DIRECTIONS

1. Take a blender, place peaches in it, and blend for 30 seconds until smooth.

2. Then add the remaining ingredients in a blender, pulse for 1 minute until combined, and then pour the smoothie into a glass.

3. Serve straight away.

PREPARATION
5 MIN

COOKING
0 MIN

SERVES FOR
1 PEOPLE

NUTRITION: calories 124, fat 12, fiber 2, carbs 25, protein 10

Pineapple Punch

INGREDIENTS

o Pineapple slices as needed for garnishing

o 8 ounces crushed pineapple

o 4 cups of pineapple juice

o 4 cups of lemon-lime soda

o 4 cups of ice cubes

DIRECTIONS

1. Take a large punch bowl, place all the ingredients in it, and stir until mixed.

2. Pour punch into glasses, add a slice of pineapple, and then serve.

PREPARATION
8 MIN

COOKING
0 MIN

SERVES FOR
2 PEOPLE

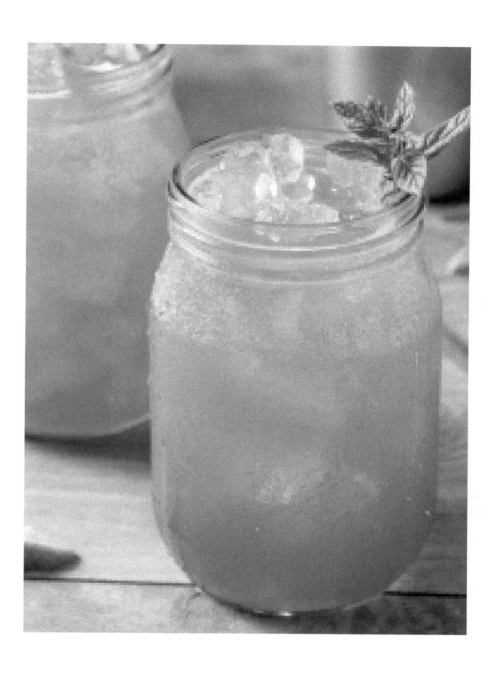

NUTRITION: calories 224, fat 12, fiber 5, carbs 15, protein 5

Citrus Shake

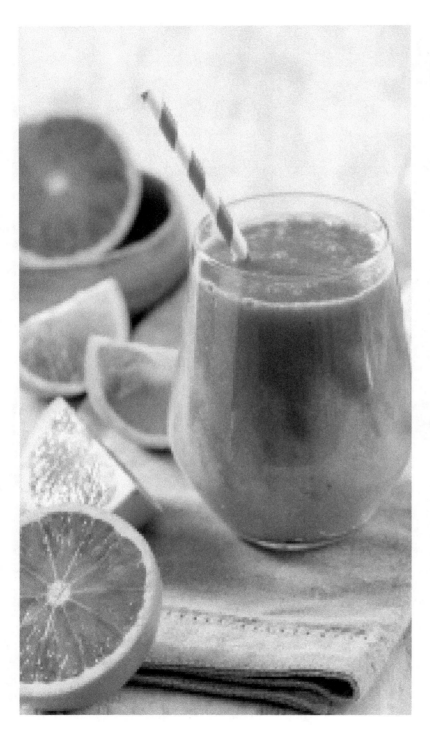

INGREDIENTS

o   1/2 cup of pineapple juice

o   1/2 cup of almond milk, unsweetened

o   1 cup of orange sherbet

o   1/2 cup of liquid egg substitute, low-cholesterol

DIRECTIONS

1. Take a blender, place all the ingredients (in order) in it, and then process for 30 seconds until smooth.

2. Distribute the shake between two glasses and then serve.

PREPARATION
10 MIN

COOKING
50 MIN

SERVES FOR
2 PEOPLE

NUTRITION: calories 124, fat 12, fiber 5, carbs 15, protein 6

Apple Smoothie

INGREDIENTS

- o 2 cups shredded kale
- o 1 cup of unsweetened almond milk
- o 1/4 cup 2 percent plain Greek yogurt
- o 1/2 Granny Smith apple, unpeeled, cored, and chopped
- o 1/2 avocado, diced
- o 3 ice cubes

DIRECTIONS:

1. Put all ingredients in a blender and blend until smooth and thick.

2. Pour into two glasses and serve immediately.

PREPARATION
10 MIN

COOKING
0 MIN

SERVES FOR
2 PEOPLE

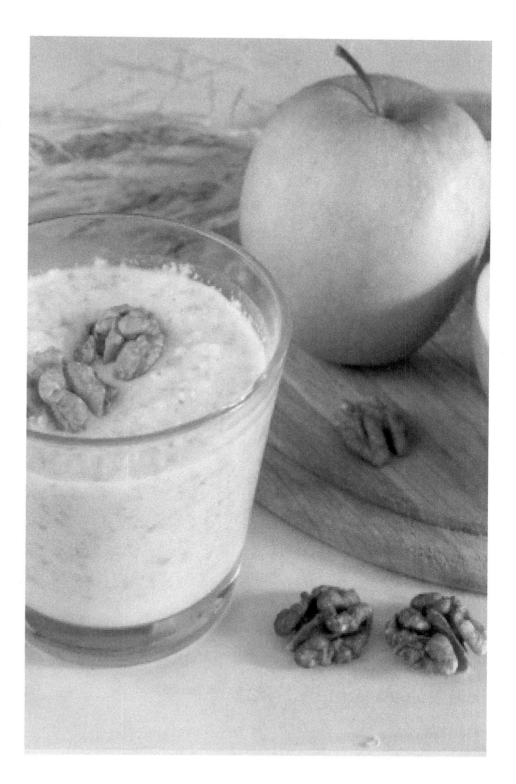

NUTRITION: calories 120, fat 2, fiber 4, carbs 27, protein 2

Broccoli Cucumber Smoothie

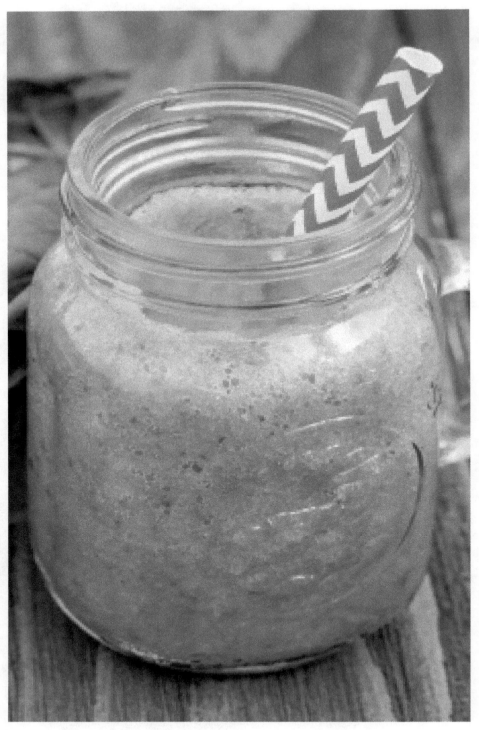

INGREDIENTS

o 1/2 medium cucumber, make slices

o 1 celery stalk, diced

o 1/2 cup of broccoli florets

o Coconut water as needed

DIRECTIONS

1. Take your blender or processor; add the cucumber, celery, broccoli, and coconut water one by one.

2. Blend or process all the ingredients for 15-20 seconds to combine well and make a smooth mixture. (If using a processor, process over high-speed setting.)

3. Pour this fresh smoothie mixture into a serving glass.

Enjoy your fresh smoothie!

PREPARATION
10 MIN

COOKING
0 MIN

SERVES FOR
2 PEOPLE

NUTRITION: calories 120, fat 2, fiber 4, carbs 27, protein 2

Cucumber Smoothie

INGREDIENTS

- o 1/2 medium cucumber, diced
- o 1 handful kale, torn
- o 2 tbs. of lemon juice
- o 1 tsp. of maple syrup

DIRECTIONS:

1. Take your blender or processor; add the kale, cucumber, lemon juice, maple syrup, and water one by one.

2. Blend or process all the ingredients for 15-20 seconds to combine well, and make a smooth mixture. (If using a processor, process over high-speed setting.)

3. Pour this fresh smoothie mixture into a serving glass.

4. Top with a slice of cucumber or lemon.

Enjoy your fresh smoothie!

PREPARATION
10 MIN

COOKING
0 MIN

SERVES FOR
2 PEOPLE

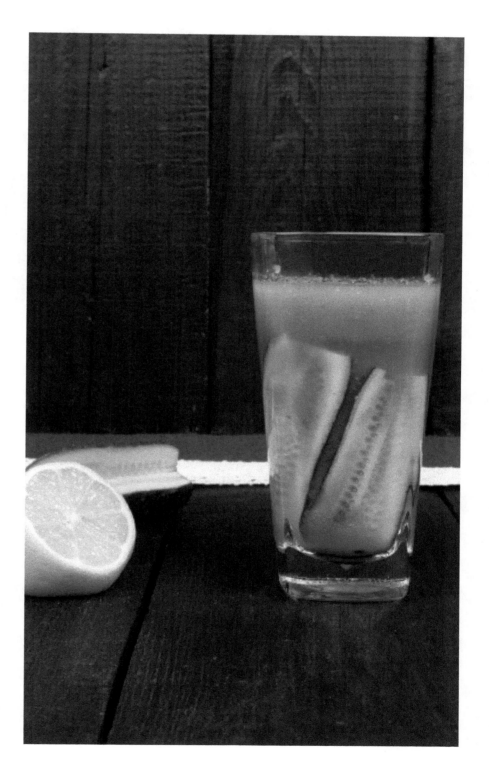

NUTRITION: calories 120, fat 2, fiber 4, carbs 27, protein 2

Spinach Tomato Smoothie

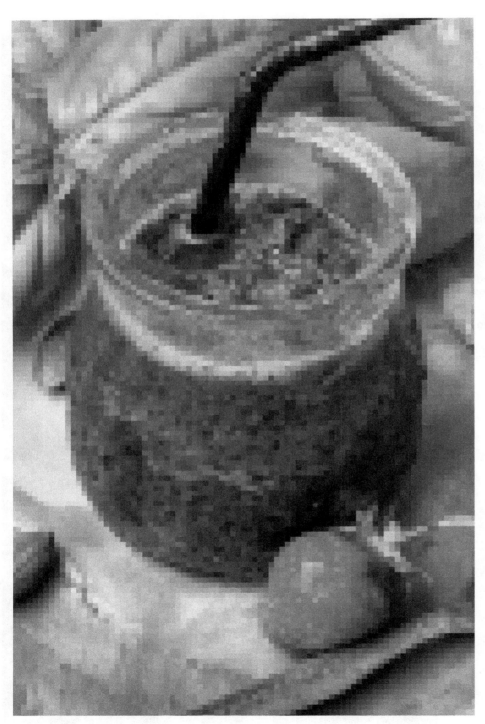

INGREDIENTS

o   1 carrot, chopped

o   1/2 celery rib, chopped

o   1/2 cup of chopped spinach

o   3 tomatoes, make halves

o   1/2 cup of mint leaves

DIRECTIONS

1. Take your blender or processor; one by one add the smoothie ingredients.

2. Blend or process the ingredients for 20-30 seconds to combine well and make a smooth mixture. (If using a processor, process over high-speed setting.)

3. Pour this fresh smoothie mixture into a serving glass.

Enjoy your fresh smoothie!

PREPARATION
10 MIN

COOKING
0 MIN

SERVES FOR
2 PEOPLE

NUTRITION: calories 120, fat 2, fiber 4, carbs 27, protein 2

Tropical Smoothie

INGREDIENTS

- 1 big piece of Mango
- 1 cup of Pineapple
- 2 handful of Kale
- Half cup of Orange

DIRECTIONS

1. Remove the seeds from the orange and peel it properly.
2. Place all the ingredients in your blender and turn it on.

PREPARATION
10 MIN

COOKING
0 MIN

SERVES FOR
2 PEOPLE

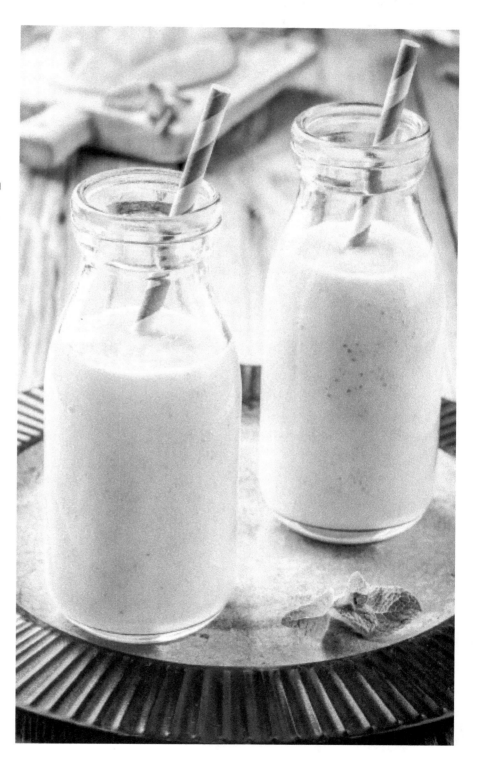

NUTRITION: calories 120, fat 2, fiber 4, carbs 27, protein 2

Blueberry Avocado Smoothie

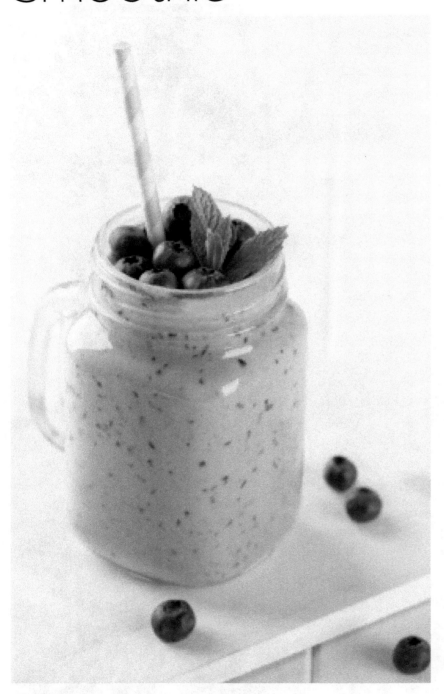

INGREDIENTS

o 1/2 cup of blueberries

o 1 tsp chia seeds

o 1/2 cup of unsweetened coconut milk

o 1 avocado

DIRECTIONS:

1. Soak chia seed in water for overnight.

2. Add all ingredients into the blender and blend until smooth and creamy.

Serve and enjoy.

PREPARATION
10 MIN

COOKING
0 MIN

SERVES FOR
2 PEOPLE

NUTRITION: calories 120, fat 2, fiber 4, carbs 27, protein 2

Mix Berry Watermelon Smoothie

INGREDIENTS

o   1 1/2 cups mixed berries

o   2 cups of watermelon

o   1 cup of coconut water

o   2 fresh lemon juices

o   1/4 cup of fresh mint leaves

DIRECTIONS:

1. Add all ingredients into the blender and blend until smooth and creamy.

Serve and enjoy.

PREPARATION
10 MIN

COOKING
0 MIN

SERVES FOR
2 PEOPLE

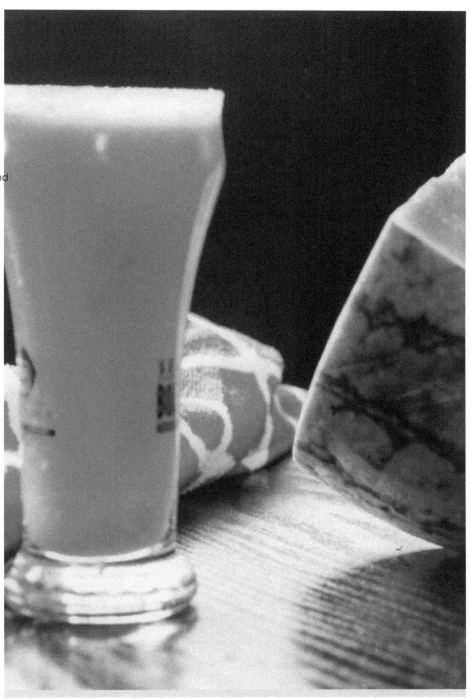

NUTRITION: calories 120, fat 2, fiber 4, carbs 27, protein 2

Blackberry Apple Smoothie

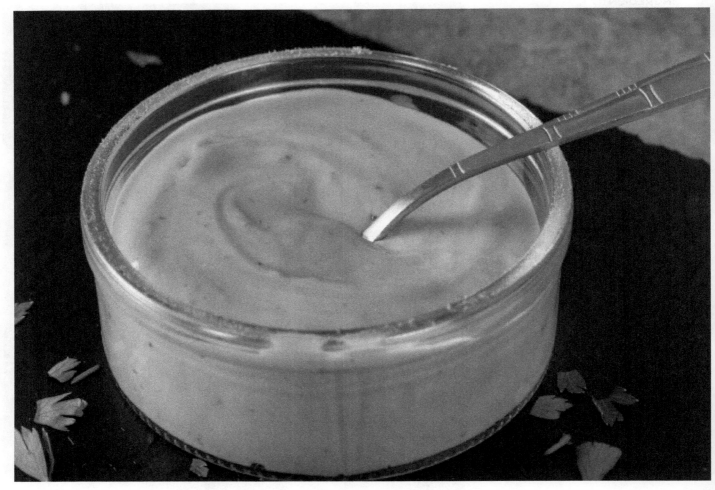

PREPARATION
10 MIN

COOKING
0 MIN

SERVES FOR
2 PEOPLE

INGREDIENTS

o   2 cups of blackberries

o   1 cup of apple juice

o   1 banana

DIRECTIONS

1.   Add all ingredients into the blender and blend until smooth and creamy.
Serve and enjoy.

NUTRITION: calories 120, fat 2, fiber 4, carbs 27, protein 2

Cranberry Blackberry Smoothie

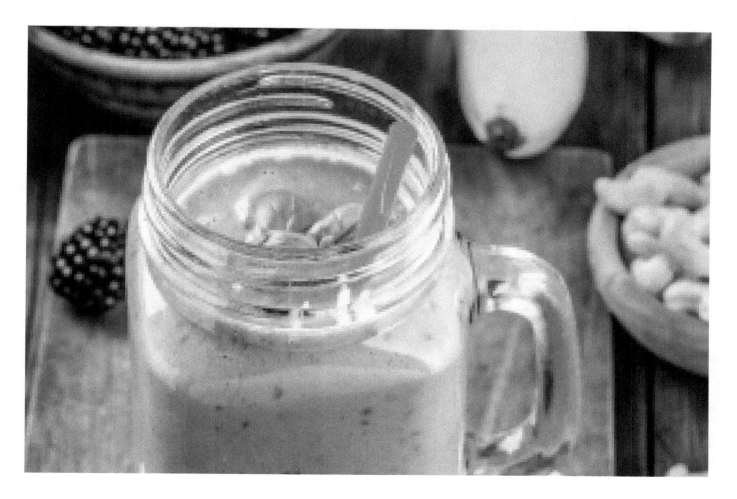

INGREDIENTS

o   1 1/2 cups of cranberries

o   1 1/2 cups of blackberries

o   1 tbsp honey

o   1 banana

DIRECTIONS

1. Add all ingredients into the blender and blend until smooth and creamy.

Serve and enjoy.

PREPARATION
10 MIN

COOKING
0 MIN

SERVES FOR
2 PEOPLE

NUTRITION: calories 120, fat 2, fiber 4, carbs 27, protein 2

Coconut Milk Smoothie

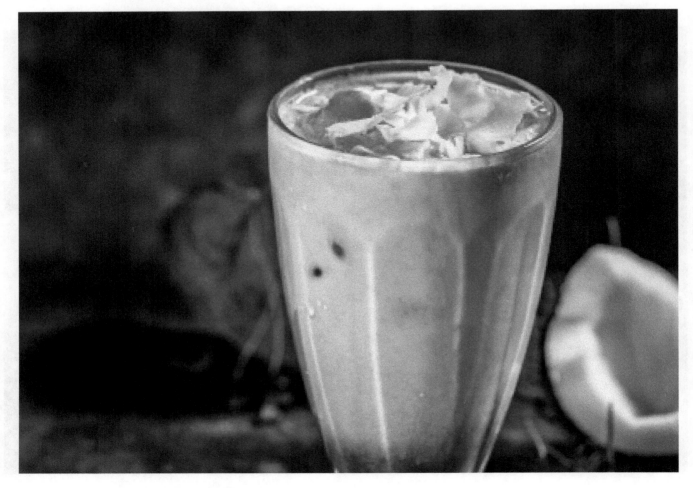

PREPARATION
10 MIN

_____

COOKING
0 MIN

SERVES FOR
2 PEOPLE

INGREDIENTS

o 1 cup of young Thai coconut meat

o 2 cups of coconut water

o 2 dates (pitted)

o 1/2 vanilla pod

DIRECTIONS

1. Place 1 cup of the coconut water in the blender.

2. You may need to strain the water if there is shell or fiber debris.

3. Remove the meat and clean to remove any shell or fibers. Take 6-8 oz (by weight) of the coconut meat and place it in the blender.

4. Blend until smooth. Store in a sealed jar. Will last 3-4 days in the fridge.

NUTRITION: calories 120, fat 2, fiber 4, carbs 27, protein 2

Sesame Cashew Nut Milk Smoothie

INGREDIENTS

o 1 cup of sesame seeds (soaked 8 hours and rinsed well)

o 1 cup of cashews (soaked 8 hours and rinsed well)

o 3 cups of filtered water - more or less depending on how creamy you like

o 4 dates (pitted)

o 1 whole vanilla bean (cut into small pieces)

DIRECTIONS

1. Add the seeds, nuts, and water.

2. Blend to break up the sesame seeds and nuts.

3. Then add the dates, vanilla, and sweetener.

4. Blend again until well liquefied. Use a nut milk bag to strain and store in a sealed jar/bottle.

5. Will last up to 3-5 days in the fridge.

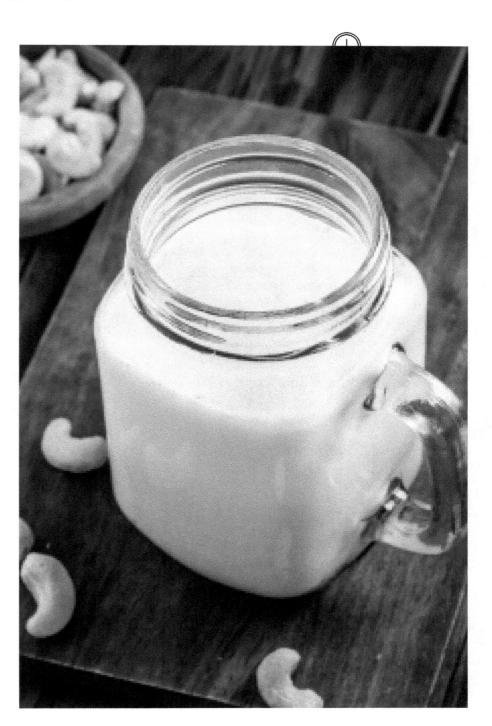

NUTRITION: calories 120, fat 2, fiber 4, carbs 27, protein 2

Almond Hemp Nut Milk Smoothie

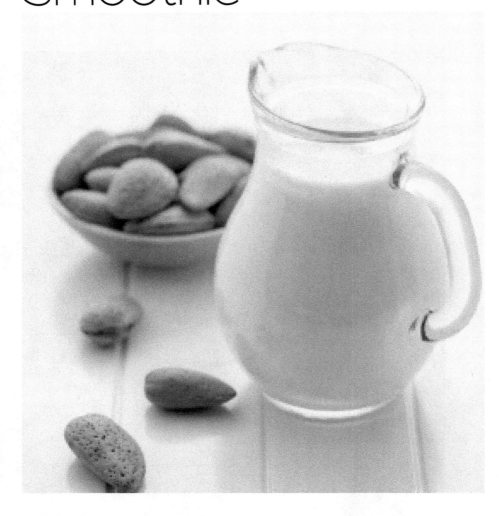

INGREDIENTS

o 1 1/2 cup of soaked almonds (overnight and rinsed well)

o 1/2 cup of hemp seed

o 3 cups of filtered water - more or less depending on how creamy you like it

o 4 dates (pitted)

o 1 vanilla pod

DIRECTIONS

1. Add nuts and water and blend. Next add the remaining ingredients and blend until liquefied.

2. Using a nut milk bag strain. Store in a sealed jar/bottle. Will keep 3-5 days in the fridge.

PREPARATION
10 MIN

COOKING
0 MIN

SERVES FOR
2 PEOPLE

NUTRITION: calories 520, fat 12, fiber 4, carbs 67, protein 9

Chapter 8: Snacks and Sides Recipes

Zucchini Pasta

INGREDIENTS

- o 3 Tablespoons of olive oil
- o 2 Cloves garlic, minced
- o 3 Zucchini, large & diced
- o Sea salt & black pepper to taste
- o 1/2 Cup of milk, 2%
- o 1/4 Teaspoon of nutmeg
- o 1 Tablespoon of lemon juice, fresh
- o 1/2 Cup of parmesan, grated
- o 8 Ounces uncooked farfalle pasta

DIRECTIONS

1. Get out a skillet and place it over medium heat, and then heat up the oil. Add in your garlic and cook for a minute. Stir often so that it doesn't burn. Add in your salt, pepper, and zucchini. Stir well, and cook covered for fifteen minutes. During this time, you'll want to stir the mixture twice.

2. Get out a microwave-safe bowl, and heat the milk for thirty seconds. Stir in your nutmeg, and then pour it into the skillet. Cook uncovered for five minutes. Stir occasionally to keep from burning.

3. Get out a stockpot and cook your pasta per package instructions. Drain the pasta, and then save two tablespoons of pasta water.

4. Stir everything together, and add in the cheese, and lemon juice and pasta water.

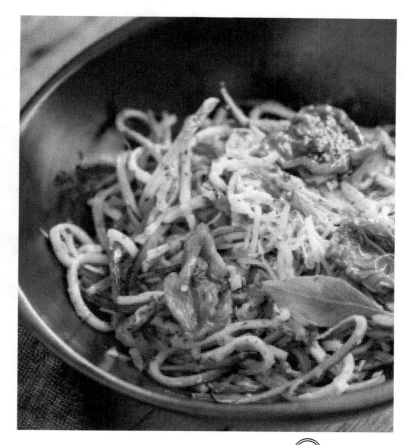

PREPARATION
15 MIN

COOKING
30 MIN

SERVES FOR
4 PEOPLE

NUTRITION: calories 414, fat 12, fiber 2, carbs 45, protein 15

Feta & Spinach Pita Bake

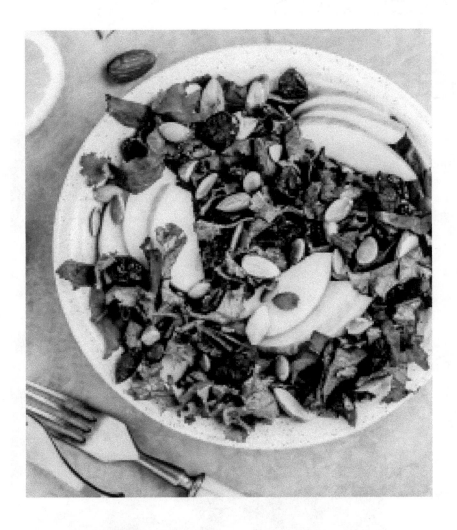

INGREDIENTS

- o 2 Roma tomatoes, chopped
- o 6 Whole wheat Pita bread
- o 1 Jar sun dried tomato pesto
- o 4 Mushrooms, fresh & sliced
- o 1 Bunch spinach, rinsed & chopped
- o 2 Tablespoons Parmesan cheese, grated
- o 3 Tablespoons olive oil
- o 1/2 Cup of Feta cheese, crumbled
- o Dash black pepper

DIRECTIONS

1. Start by heating the oven to 350, and get to your pita bread. Spread the tomato pesto on the side of each one. Put them in a baking pan with the tomato side up.

2. Top with tomatoes, spinach, mushrooms, parmesan, and feta. Drizzle with olive oil and season with pepper.

3. Bake for twelve minutes, and then serve cut into quarters.

PREPARATION
10 MIN

COOKING
20 MIN

SERVES FOR
6 PEOPLE

NUTRITION: calories 324, fat 12, fiber 4, carbs 34, protein 15

Cranberries Spring Salad

INGREDIENTS

- o 1/2 cup of cooked lentils
- o 1/2 cup of finely chopped arugula
- o 1/2 cucumber, sliced
- o 1/2 orange, peeled and sectioned
- o 1/2 carrot, sliced
- o 1/2 green bell pepper, sliced
- o 1/4 cup of fresh cranberries
- o 1/4 cup of olive oil
- o 1/2 tsp of ground red pepper
- o 1/4 tsp of salt
- o 1 tsp of balsamic vinegar

DIRECTIONS

1. Combine the vegetables in a large bowl. Add lentils and mix well. Set aside.

2. In a smaller bowl, shake together the balsamic vinegar, olive oil, salt, and red pepper. Put the vinaigrette over the vegetables and mix well. Top with orange and cranberries.

Serve cold.

PREPARATION
15 MIN

COOKING
0 MIN

SERVES FOR
2 PEOPLE

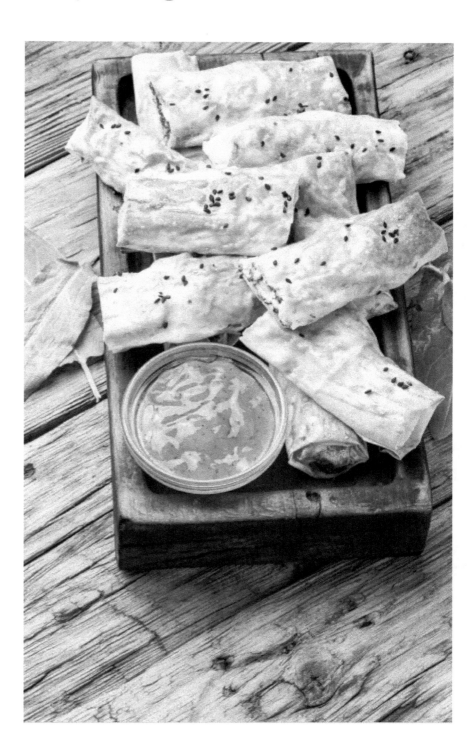

NUTRITION: Calories 194 Fat 26 Carbs 41 Protein 32

Veggie Fritters

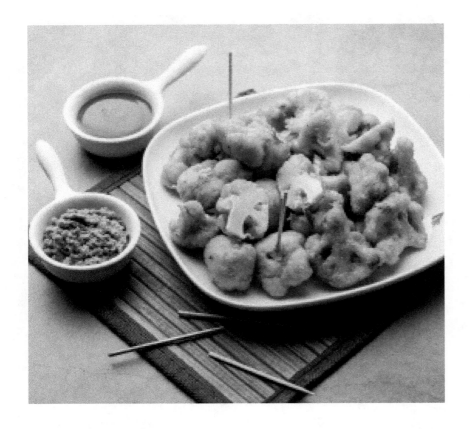

INGREDIENTS

- o 2 garlic cloves, minced
- o 2 yellow onions, chopped
- o 4 scallions, chopped
- o 2 carrots, grated
- o 2 teaspoons cumin, ground
- o 1/2 teaspoon of turmeric powder
- o Salt and black pepper to the taste
- o 1/4 teaspoon of coriander, ground
- o 2 tablespoons of parsley, chopped
- o 1/4 teaspoon of lemon juice
- o 1/2 cup of almond flour
- o 2 beets, peeled and grated
- o 2 eggs, whisked
- o 1/4 cup of tapioca flour
- o 3 tablespoons of olive oil

DIRECTIONS:

1. In a bowl, combine the garlic with the onions, scallions, and the rest of the ingredients except the oil, stir well and shape medium fritters out of this mix.

2. Heat up a pan with the oil over medium-high heat, add the fritters, cook for 5 minutes on each side, arrange on a platter, and serve.

PREPARATION
10 MIN

COOKING
10 MIN

SERVES FOR
8 PEOPLE

NUTRITION: calories 204, fat 11, fiber 3, carbs 15, protein 48

Cucumber Bites

INGREDIENTS

- o 1 English cucumber, sliced into 32 rounds
- o 10 ounces hummus
- o 16 cherry tomatoes, halved
- o 1 tablespoon of parsley, chopped
- o 1 ounce feta cheese, crumbled

DIRECTIONS

1. Spread the hummus on each cucumber round, divide the tomato halves on each, sprinkle the cheese and parsley on to, and serve as an appetizer.

PREPARATION
10 MIN

COOKING
0 MIN

SERVES FOR
12 PEOPLE

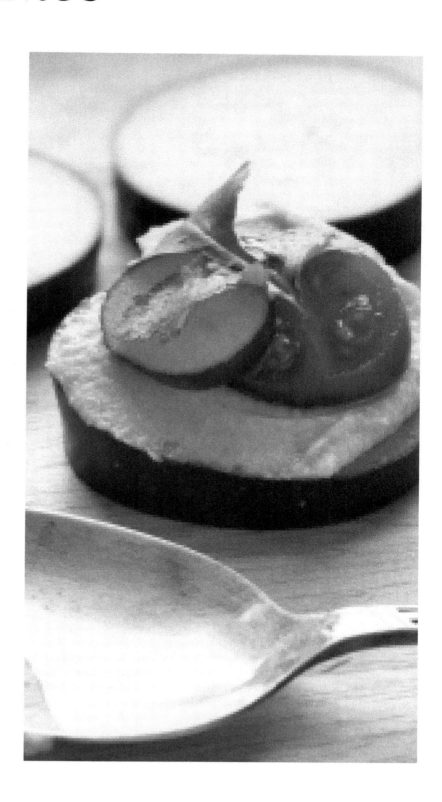

NUTRITION: Calories 162; Fat 3.4; Fiber 2; Carbs 6.4; Protein 2.4

Artichoke Flatbread

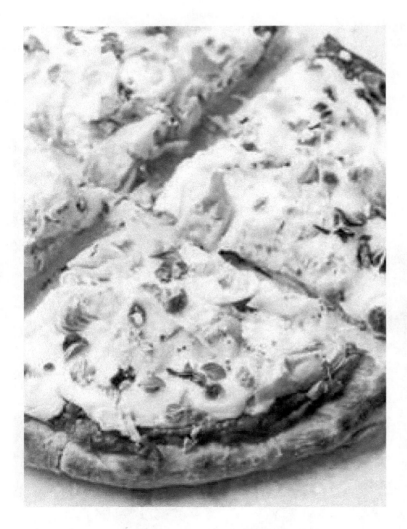

INGREDIENTS

- o 5 tablespoons olive oil
- o 2 garlic cloves, minced
- o 2 tablespoons parsley, chopped
- o 2 round whole wheat flatbreads
- o 4 tablespoons parmesan, grated
- o 1/2 cup mozzarella cheese, grated
- o 14 ounces canned artichokes, drained and quartered
- o 1 cup baby spinach, chopped
- o 1/2 cup cherry tomatoes, halved
- o 1/2 teaspoon basil, dried
- o Salt and black pepper to the taste

DIRECTIONS

1. In a bowl, mix the parsley with the garlic and 4 tablespoons oil, whisk well, and spread this over the flatbreads.

2. Sprinkle the mozzarella and half of the parmesan.

3. In a bowl, mix the artichokes with the spinach, tomatoes, basil, salt, pepper, and the rest of the oil, toss and divide over the flatbreads as well.

4. Sprinkle the rest of the parmesan on top, arrange the flatbreads on a baking sheet lined with parchment paper and bake at 425° F for 15 minutes.

Serve as an appetizer.

PREPARATION
10 MIN

COOKING
15 MIN

SERVES FOR
4 PEOPLE

NUTRITION: calories 224, fat 11, fiber 5, carbs 15, protein 8

Red Pepper Tapenade

INGREDIENTS

- o 7 ounces roasted red peppers, chopped
- o 1/2 cup parmesan, grated
- o 1/3 cup parsley, chopped
- o 14 ounces canned artichokes, drained and chopped
- o 3 tablespoons olive oil
- o 1/4 cup capers, drained
- o 1 and 1/2 tablespoons lemon juice
- o 2 garlic cloves, minced

DIRECTIONS

1. In your blender, combine the red peppers with the parmesan and the rest of the ingredients and pulse well.

2. Divide into cups and serve as a snack.

PREPARATION
10 MIN

COOKING
10 MIN

SERVES FOR
4 PEOPLE

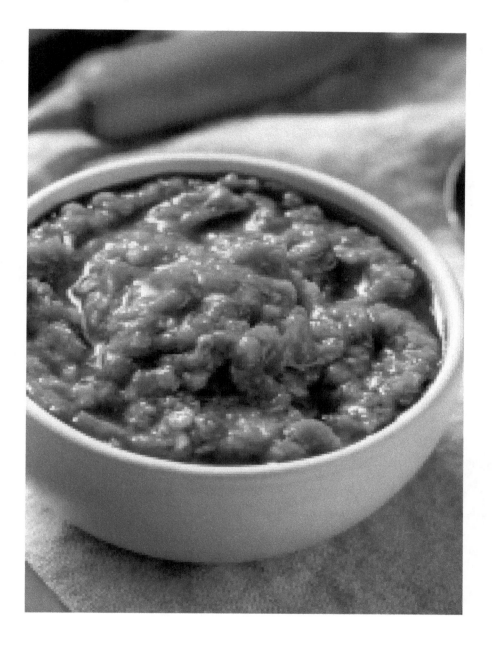

NUTRITION: calories 200, fat 6, fiber 5, carbs 13, protein 7

Coriander Falafel

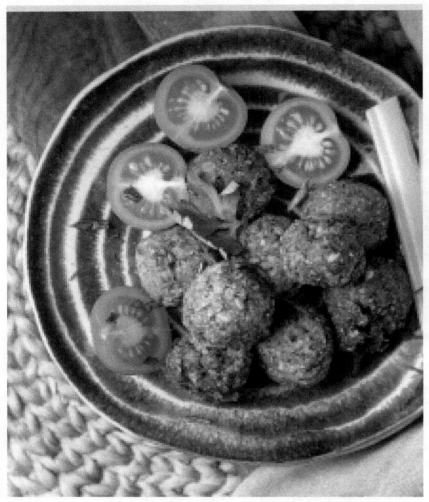

INGREDIENTS

o 1 cup canned garbanzo beans, drained and rinsed

o 1 bunch parsley leaves

o 1 yellow onion, chopped

o 5 garlic cloves, minced

o 1 teaspoon coriander, ground

o A pinch of salt and black pepper

o 1/4 teaspoon cayenne pepper

o 1/4 teaspoon baking soda

o 1/4 teaspoon cumin powder

o 1 teaspoon lemon juice

o 3 tablespoons tapioca flour

o Olive oil for frying

DIRECTIONS

1. In your food processor, combine the beans with the parsley, onion, and the rest of the ingredients except the oil and the flour and pulse well.

2. Transfer the mix to a bowl, add the flour, stir well, shape 16 balls out of this mix and flatten them a bit.

3. Heat up a pan with some oil over medium-high heat, add the falafels, cook them for 5 minutes on each side, transfer to paper towels, drain excess grease, arrange them on a platter and serve as an appetizer.

PREPARATION
10 MIN

COOKING
10 MIN

SERVES FOR
8 PEOPLE

NUTRITION: Calories 112; Fat 6.2; Fiber 2; Carbs 12.3; Protein 3.1

Red Pepper Hummus

INGREDIENTS

- 6 ounces roasted red peppers, peeled and chopped
- 16 ounces canned chickpeas, drained and rinsed
- 1/4 cup Greek yogurt
- 3 tablespoons tahini paste
- Juice of 1 lemon
- 3 garlic cloves, minced
- 1 tablespoon olive oil
- A pinch of salt and black pepper
- 1 tablespoon parsley, chopped

DIRECTIONS:

1. In your food processor, combine the red peppers with the rest of the ingredients except the oil and the parsley and pulse well.

2. Add the oil, pulse again, divide into cups, sprinkle the parsley on top, and serve as a party spread.

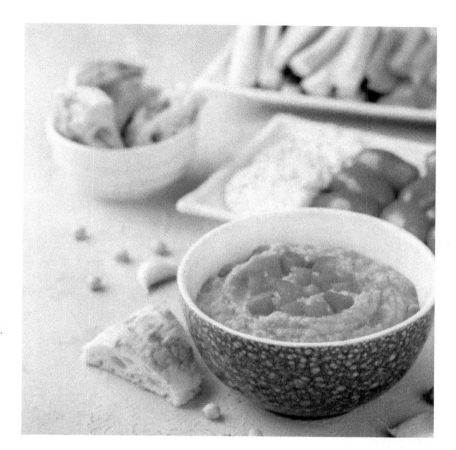

NUTRITION: calories 254, fat 12, fiber 5, carbs 17, protein 5

Mint Labneh

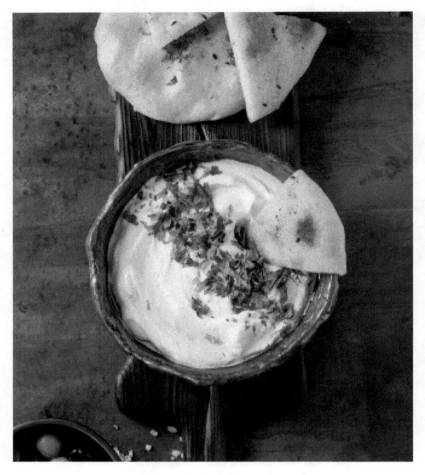

INGREDIENTS

o   32 ounces Plain Yogurt, or store-bought

o   1/2 teaspoon salt

o   1/4 cup olive oil

o   1/4 cup finely chopped fresh mint

DIRECTIONS

1.   Stir together the yogurt and salt.

2.   Put a colander with some layers of cheesecloth. Put some of the yogurt mixture into the lined colander. Place the colander over a sink or a bowl and let the mixture sit for 2 hours just until most of the water is drained.

3.   Spoon the labneh into a small bowl and stir in the olive oil and mint until well combined. The labneh can be refrigerated in an airtight container for 1 to 2 weeks.

PREPARATION
10 MIN

COOKING
0 MIN

SERVES FOR
6 PEOPLE

Sweet and Sour Beet Dip

INGREDIENTS

- o 1-pound beets, trimmed
- o 1/2 cup tahini
- o 1/2 cup freshly squeezed lemon juice
- o 4 garlic cloves, mashed
- o Grated zest of 1 lemon
- o 1 teaspoon ground cumin
- o 1/4 teaspoon cayenne pepper
- o Salt
- o Freshly ground black pepper

DIRECTIONS:

1. Mix the beets with enough water and then cover. Place the pan on high heat and boil the beets for about 50 minutes or until tender.

2. Drain the beets, let them cool, and peel them. The skins should slide off easily.

3. Transfer the beets to a food processor and purée for about 5 minutes until smooth. Transfer the puréed beets to a medium bowl.

4. Stir in the tahini, lemon juice, garlic, lemon zest, cumin, and cayenne until well mixed. Taste and then season it with some salt and black pepper, as needed.

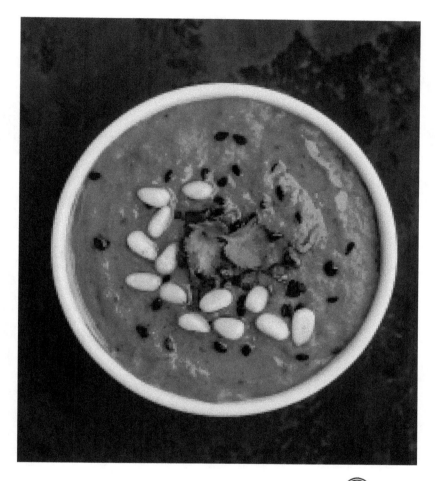

PREPARATION
10 MIN

COOKING
50 MIN

SERVES FOR
6 PEOPLE

NUTRITION: calories 162, fat 11, fiber 4, carbs 13, protein 4

Marinated Olives

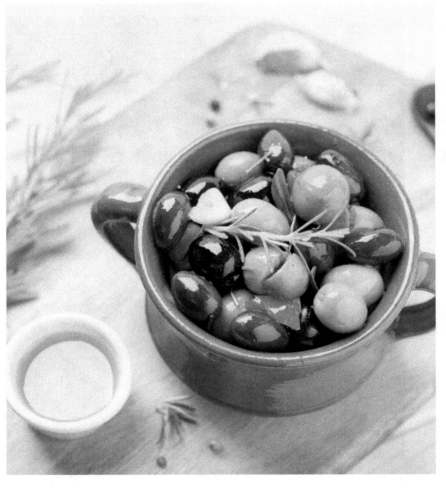

INGREDIENTS

o 1/4 cup olive oil

o 1/4 cup red wine vinegar

o Grated zest of 1 lemon

o 1 teaspoon chopped fresh rosemary

o 2 cups jarred olives, drained

DIRECTIONS:

1. Whisk the olive oil, vinegar, lemon zest, and rosemary until blended.

2. Add the olives and gently stir to coat. Put well and let it marinate for at least 3 hours before serving.

PREPARATION
10 MIN

COOKING
0 MIN

SERVES FOR
4 PEOPLE

NUTRITION: calories 204, fat 21, fiber 3, carbs 7, protein 1

Marinated Zucchini

INGREDIENTS

- o 1/4 cup balsamic vinegar
- o 2 tablespoons stone-ground mustard
- o 1 garlic clove, minced
- o 2 teaspoons chopped fresh thyme
- o 1/4 cup olive oil
- o 1/8 teaspoon salt
- o 1/8 teaspoon freshly ground black pepper
- o 3 large zucchinis, cut diagonally into 1/2-inch-thick slices

DIRECTIONS:

1. Whisk the vinegar, mustard, garlic, and thyme to combine. Whisk in the olive oil until blended. Season with the salt and pepper and whisk again to combine.

2. Place the zucchini in a large bowl and drizzle 1/4 cup of marinade over them. Toss well to coat.

3. Heat a grill pan or sauté pan over medium heat.

4. Transfer the cooked zucchini back to the bowl and drizzle it with the remaining marinade. Toss to coat. Cover the bowl and refrigerate the zucchini to marinate for 30 minutes or until chilled.

5. Arrange the marinated slices on a serving platter and drizzle with the marinade from the bowl to serve.

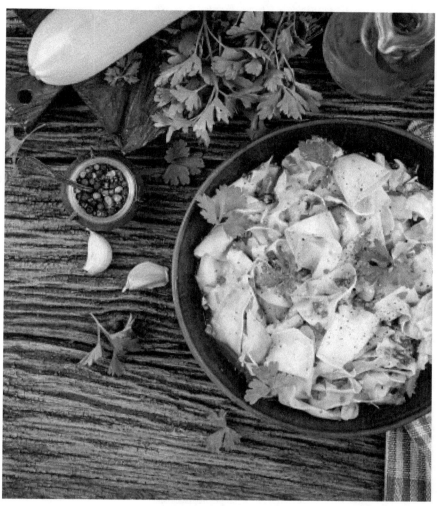

PREPARATION
15 MIN

COOKING
5 MIN

SERVES FOR
6 PEOPLE

NUTRITION: calories 104, fat 8, fiber 2, carbs 5, protein 2

Pickled Turnips

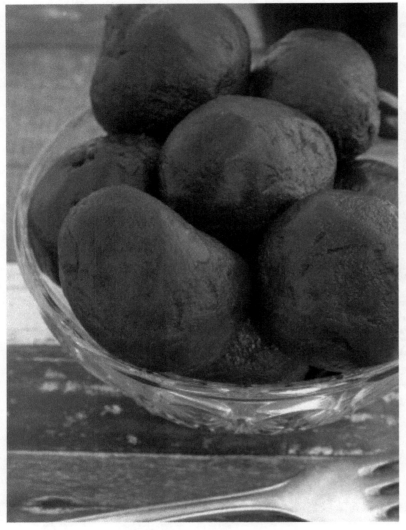

INGREDIENTS

o 4 cups of water

o 1/4 cup of salt

o 1 cup of white distilled vinegar

o 1 small beet, peeled and quartered

o 1 garlic clove, peeled

o 2 pounds turnips, peeled, halved, and cut into 1/4-inch half-moons

DIRECTIONS:

1. In a medium bowl, whisk the water and salt until the salt dissolves. Whisk in the vinegar.

2. Place the beet and garlic in a clean 2-quart glass jar with a tight-sealing lid. Layer the turnips on top.

3. Pour the vinegar mixture over the turnips to cover them. Seal the lid tightly and let the jar sit at room temperature for 1 week.

PREPARATION
15 MIN

COOKING
0 MIN

SERVES FOR
12 PEOPLE

NUTRITION: calories 24, fat 0, fiber 1, carbs 15, protein 1

Chapter 9: Soups and stews Recipes

Roasted Pork Soup

INGREDIENTS

- o 3 cups mixed vegetables
- o 2 tbsp ginger and garlic, minced
- o Salt and pepper
- o 1 cup roasted pork cubes
- o 3 cups vegetable broth

DIRECTIONS:

1. Put all the ingredients (except pork) in the instant pot cooker and lock the lid. Cook with Soup setting for 10 minutes and then let the pressure release naturally.

2. Now, add the roasted pork cubes and stir the soup thoroughly and cook for another 5 minutes without the lid to get the right consistency of the soup.

Serve hot by seasoning with some more pepper and salt.

TOTAL TIME
25 MIN

SERVES FOR
4 PEOPLE

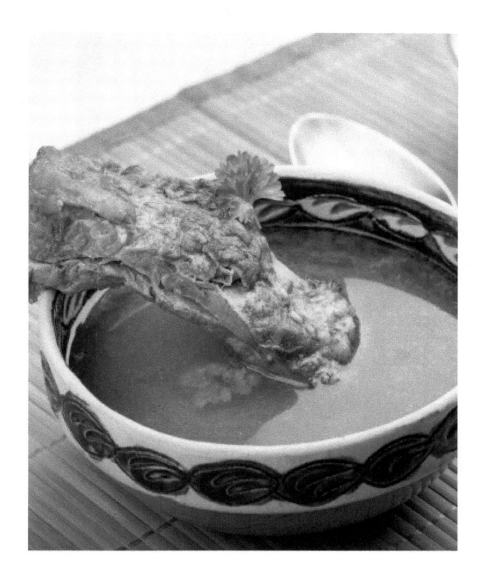

NUTRITION: calories 224, fat 12, fiber 5, carbs 15, protein 5

Roasted Red Pepper Soup

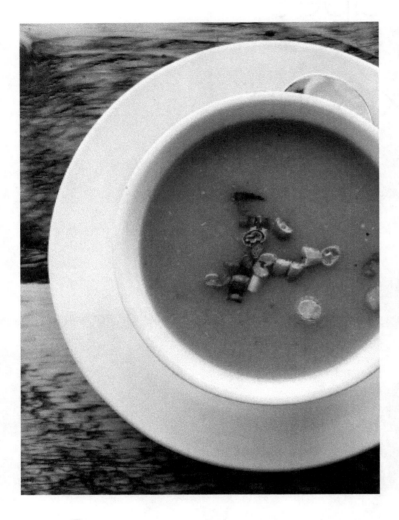

INGREDIENTS

o 4 cups low-sodium chicken broth

o 3 red peppers

o 2 medium onions

o 3 tbsp. lemon juice

o 1 tbsp. finely minced lemon zest

o A pinch of cayenne pepper

o 1/4 tsp. cinnamon

o 1/2 cup finely minced fresh cilantro

DIRECTIONS:

1. In a medium stockpot, consolidate each one of the fixings except for the cilantro and warmth to the point of boiling over excessive warm temperature.

2. Diminish the warmth and stew, ordinarily secured, for around 30 minutes, till thickened.

3. Cool marginally. Utilizing a hand blender or nourishment processor, puree the soup.

4. Include the cilantro and tenderly heat.

PREPARATION
30 MIN

COOKING
35 MIN

SERVES FOR
4 PEOPLE

NUTRITION: calories 264, fat 8, fiber 5, carbs 5, protein 25

Vegetable Confetti Relish Stew

INGREDIENTS

o 1/2 red bell pepper

o 1/2 green pepper, boiled and chopped

o 4 scallions, thinly sliced

o 1/2 tsp. ground cumin

o 3 tbsp. vegetable oil

o 1 1/2 tbsp. white wine vinegar

o black pepper to taste

DIRECTIONS:

1. Join all fixings and blend well. Chill in the fridge.

2. You can include a large portion of slashed jalapeno pepper for an increasingly fiery blend

PREPARATION
25 MIN

COOKING
15 MIN

SERVES FOR
1 PEOPLE

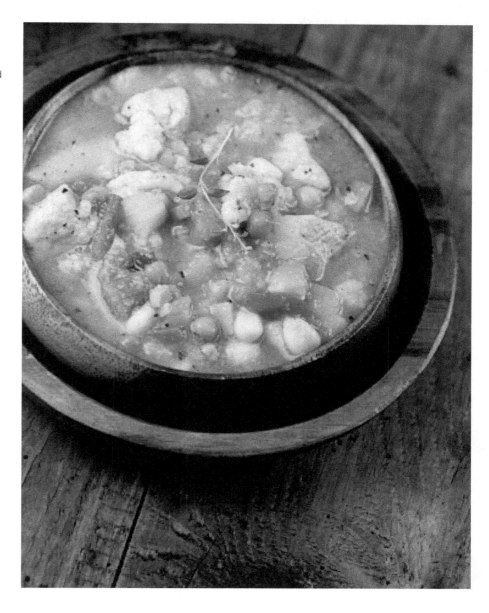

NUTRITION: calories 624, fat 22, fiber 5, carbs 25, protein 43

Mixed Lentil Stew

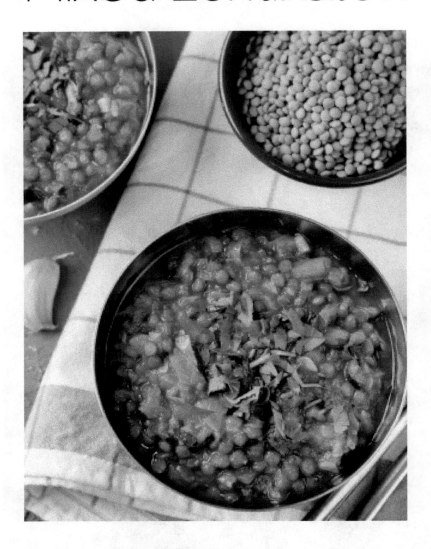

PREPARATION
10 MIN

COOKING
30 MIN

SERVES FOR
4 PEOPLE

INGREDIENTS

o   1 1/2 cups mixed lentils, rinsed

o   1/4 cup fresh cilantro, chopped

o   12 oz can chickpeas, drained and rinsed

o   1 tsp dried oregano

o   1 tsp ground sumac

o   1 tsp ground ginger

o   1 tsp garlic powder

o   1 tbsp ground cumin

o   1 tbsp paprika

o   28 oz can tomato, diced

o   2 zucchinis, chopped

o   1 bell pepper, chopped

o   3 carrots, chopped

o   1 sweet potato, chopped

o   1 onion, chopped

o   4 1/2 cups vegetable broth

o   Pepper

o   Salt

DIRECTIONS:

1. Add all ingredients except chickpeas and cilantro into the inner pot of instant pot and stir well.

2. Seal pot with lid and cook on high for minutes.

3. Once done, release pressure using quick release. Remove lid.

4. Add cilantro and chickpeas and stir well.

Serve and enjoy.

NUTRITION: calories 524, fat 5, fiber 5, carbs 10, protein 20

Creamy Potato Soup

INGREDIENTS

o 3/4 lbs. potato, peeled and diced

o 2 leeks, sliced

o 4 cups vegetable stock

o 1 tsp garlic, minced

o 1 onion, chopped

o 1 tbsp olive oil

o Pepper

o Salt

DIRECTIONS:

1. Add oil into the inner pot of instant pot and set the pot on sauté mode.

2. Add onion and sauté for 2 minutes.

3. Add garlic and leek and sauté for 2 minutes.

4. Add remaining ingredients and stir well.

5. Seal pot with lid and cook on high for 6 minutes.

6. Once done, allow to release pressure naturally for 10 minutes then release remaining using quick release. Remove lid.

7. Blend soup using an immersion blender until smooth.

Serve and enjoy.

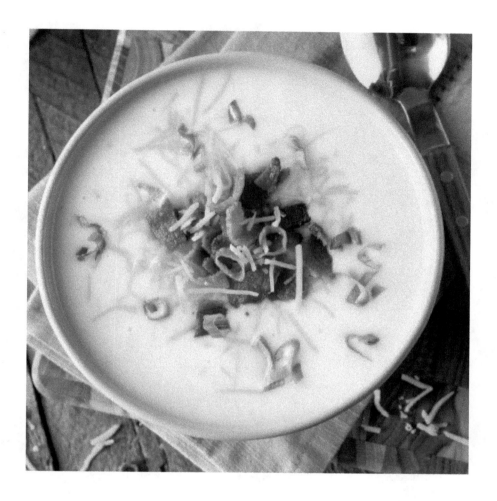

PREPARATION
10 MIN

COOKING
10 MIN

SERVES FOR
4 PEOPLE

NUTRITION: calories 144, fat 12, fiber 5, carbs 25, protein 4

Healthy Carrot Soup

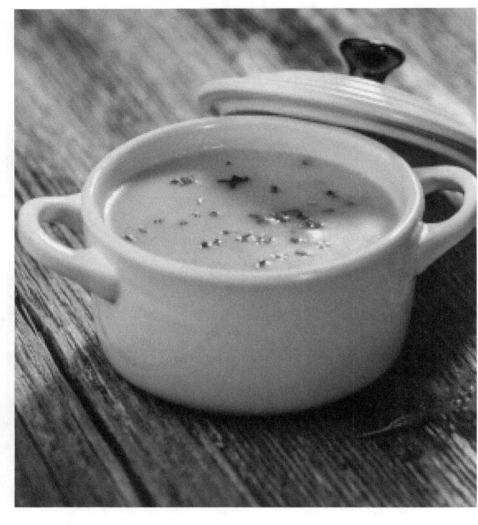

INGREDIENTS

o 1 3/4 lbs. carrots, chopped

o 1 tsp coriander powder

o 1 onion, chopped

o 1 tbsp olive oil

o 4 cups vegetable stock

o 1/4 cup fresh coriander, chopped

o Pepper

o Salt

DIRECTIONS:

1. Add oil into the inner pot of instant pot and set the pot on sauté mode.

2. Add onion and sauté until onion is softened.

3. Add remaining ingredients and stir well.

4. Seal pot with lid and cook on high for 5 minutes.

5. Once done, allow to release pressure naturally for 10 minutes then release remaining using quick release. Remove lid.

6. Blend soup using an immersion blender until smooth.

Serve and enjoy.

PREPARATION
10 MIN

COOKING
10 MIN

SERVES FOR
4 PEOPLE

NUTRITION: calories 129, fat 12, fiber 5, carbs 25, protein 3

Creamy Squash Cauliflower Soup

INGREDIENTS

- o 1 cauliflower head, cut into florets
- o 1 bell pepper, diced
- o 1 small butternut squash, peeled and chopped
- o 1/2 tsp dried parsley
- o 1/2 tsp dried mixed herbs
- o 1 cup vegetable stock
- o 1/4 cup yogurt
- o 1 onion, chopped
- o Pepper
- o Salt

DIRECTIONS:

1. Add all ingredients except yogurt into the instant pot.
2. Seal pot with lid and cook on high for 8 minutes.
3. Once done, release pressure using quick release. Remove lid.
4. Stir in yogurt and blend soup using an immersion blender until smooth.

Serve and enjoy.

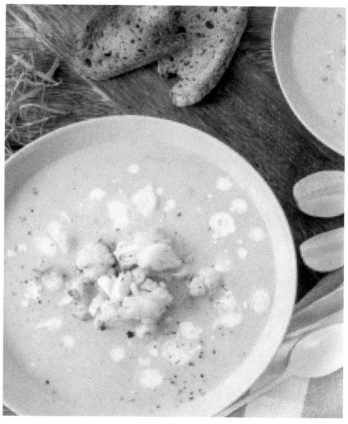

PREPARATION
10 MIN

COOKING
8 MIN

SERVES FOR
6 PEOPLE

NUTRITION: calories 224, fat 12, fiber 5, carbs 15, protein 5

Cheese Kale Soup

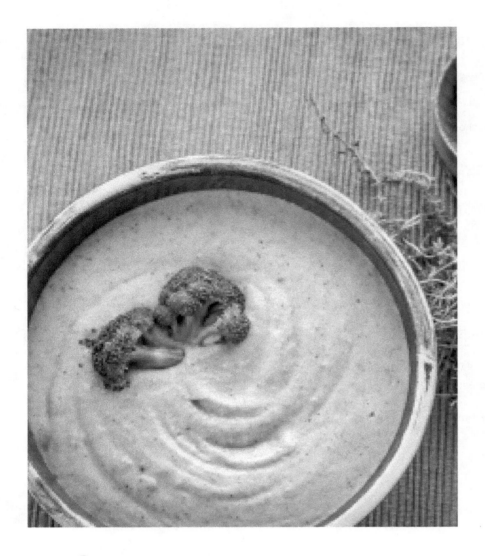

INGREDIENTS

o 6 cups fresh kale, chopped

o 1 tbsp olive oil

o 3/4 cup cottage cheese, cut into chunks

o 3 cups vegetable broth

o Pepper

o salt

DIRECTIONS:

1. Add all ingredients except cheese into the instant pot and stir well.

2. Seal pot with lid and cook on high for 5 minutes.

3. Once done, release pressure using quick release. Remove lid.

4. Stir in cottage cheese and serve.

PREPARATION
10 MIN

COOKING
5 MIN

SERVES FOR
4 PEOPLE

NUTRITION: calories 144, fat 6, fiber 3, carbs 13, protein 12

Chicken Kale Soup

INGREDIENTS

- o 2 cups cooked chicken, chopped
- o 12 oz kale, chopped
- o 2 tsp garlic, minced
- o 1 onion, diced
- o 4 cups vegetable broth
- o Salt

DIRECTIONS:

1. Add all ingredients into the instant pot and stir well.
2. Seal pot with lid and cook on high for 5 minutes.
3. Once done, allow to release pressure naturally for 5 minutes then release remaining using quick release. Remove lid.
4. Stir well and serve.

PREPARATION
10 MIN

COOKING
15 MIN

SERVES FOR
4 PEOPLE

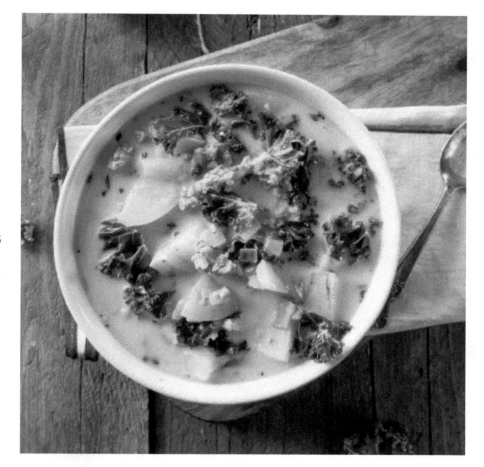

NUTRITION: calories 224, fat 12, fiber 5, carbs 15, protein 5

Cabbage Soup

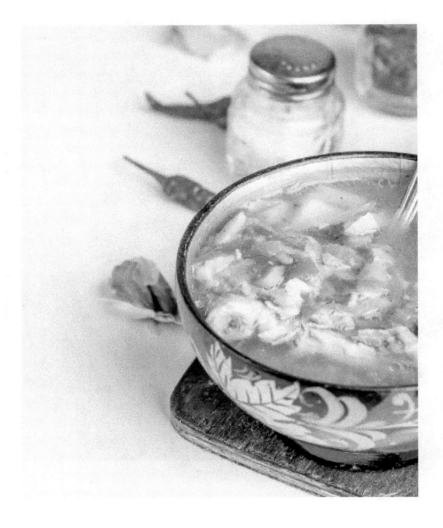

INGREDIENTS

- o 3 cups cabbage, chopped
- o 2 tbsp olive oil
- o 5 oz tomato paste
- o 14.5 oz can stewed tomatoes
- o 1/2 onion, sliced
- o 1 tbsp garlic, diced
- o 14. oz can tomato, diced
- o 4 cups vegetable stock
- o Pepper
- o Salt

DIRECTIONS

1. Add oil into the inner pot of instant pot and set the pot on sauté mode.

2. Add onion and garlic and sauté for 2 minutes.

3. Add cabbage, water, tomato paste, and tomatoes. Stir well.

4. Seal pot with lid and cook on high for 5 minutes.

5. Once done, allow to release pressure naturally for 5 minutes then release remaining using quick release. Remove lid.

Serve and enjoy.

PREPARATION
10 MIN

COOKING
7 MIN

SERVES FOR
4 PEOPLE

NUTRITION: calories 165, fat 7, fiber 3, carbs 25, protein 5

Chapter 10: Salads Recipes

Prosciutto and Figs Salad

INGREDIENTS

- o One 10-12-ounce package of fresh baby spinach
- o 1 small hot red chili pepper, finely diced
- o 1 carton figs, stems removed and quartered
- o 1/2 cup walnuts, coarsely chopped
- o 1 tablespoon fresh orange juice
- o 1 tablespoon honey
- o 4 slices prosciutto, cut into strips
- o Shaved parmesan cheese for garnish

DIRECTIONS:

1. Take your spinach and divide them into 4 equal portions. Each portion should be on a separate plate and will act as a base. Add quartered prosciutto, figs, and walnuts on each spinach as toppings.

2. For the dressing, take a small bowl and add honey, orange juice, and diced pepper. Add the mixture over the salad.

3. Finally, toss the salad lightly and use parmesan cheese for the garnish.

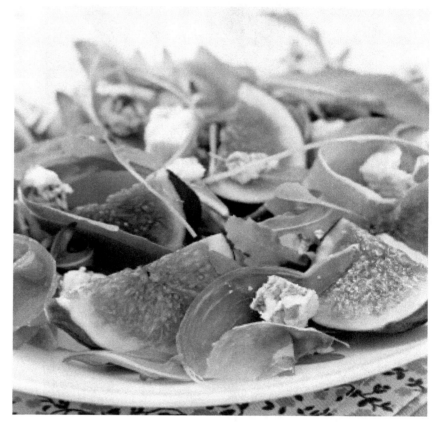

PREPARATION
10 MIN

COOKING
0 MIN

SERVES FOR
4 PEOPLE

NUTRITION: calories 190, fat 7, fiber 4, carbs 12, protein 9

Garden Vegetables and Chickpeas Salad

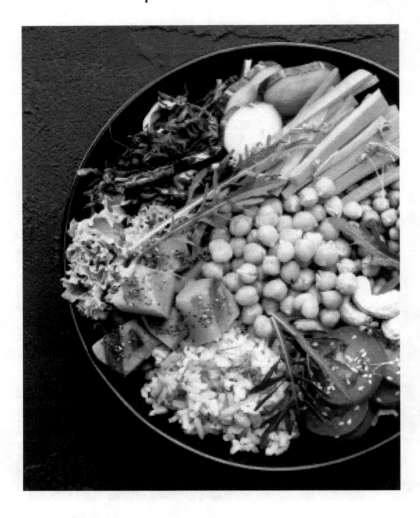

INGREDIENTS

- o 2 tablespoons freshly squeezed lemon juice
- o 1/8 Teaspoon freshly ground pepper
- o 1 cup cubed part-skim mozzarella cheese
- o 1 tablespoon fresh basil leaf, snipped
- o 1 (15-ounce) can chickpeas, rinsed and well drained
- o 2 cups coarsely chopped fresh broccoli
- o 2 cloves fresh garlic, finely minced
- o 1/2 cup sliced fresh carrots
- o 1 71/2-ounce can diced tomatoes, undrained

DIRECTIONS

1. Use a large bowl and add garlic, basil, lemon juice, and ground pepper. Mix them well.

2. Add the chickpeas, carrots, tomatoes with juice, broccoli, and mozzarella cheese. Mix all the ingredients well.

3. You can serve immediately, or you can keep it refrigerated overnight.

PREPARATION
10 MIN

COOKING
0 MIN

SERVES FOR
4 PEOPLE

NUTRITION: calories 140, fat 7, fiber 4, carbs 12, protein 4

Peppered Watercress Salad

INGREDIENTS

o 2 teaspoons champagne vinegar

o 2 bunches (about 8 cups) watercress, rinsed and rough stems removed

o 2 tablespoons extra-virgin olive oil

o Salt and freshly ground pepper to taste

DIRECTIONS:

1. Drain the watercress properly.

2. Take out a small bowl and then add salt, pepper, vinegar, and olive oil. Mix them well together.

3. Transfer the watercress to a bowl. Add the vinegar mixture into it and toss well.

Serve immediately.

PREPARATION
5 MIN

COOKING
0 MIN

SERVES FOR
4 PEOPLE

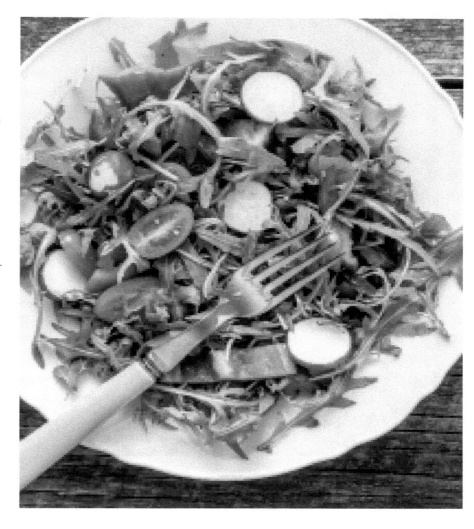

NUTRITION: calories 80, fat 7, fiber 4, carbs 1, protein 4

Broccoli Salad Moroccan Style

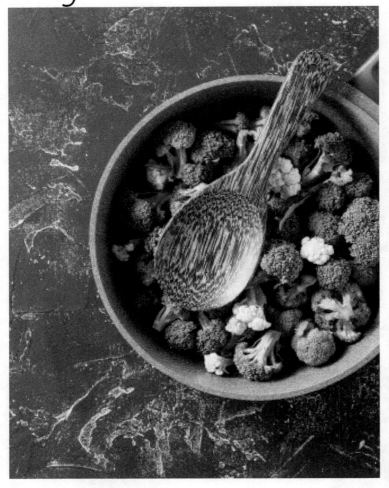

INGREDIENTS

o 1/4 tsp sea salt

o 1/4 tsp ground cinnamon

o 1/2 tsp ground turmeric

o 3/4 tsp ground ginger

o 1/2 tbsp extra virgin olive oil

o 1/2 tbsp apple cider vinegar

o 2 tbsp chopped green onion

o 1/3 cup coconut cream

o 1/2 cup carrots, shredded

o 1 small head of broccoli, chopped

DIRECTIONS:

1. In a large salad bowl, mix well salt, cinnamon, turmeric, ginger, olive oil, and vinegar.

2. Add remaining ingredients, tossing well to coat.

3. Pop in the refrigerator for at least 30 to 60 minutes before serving.

PREPARATION
20 MIN

COOKING
0 MIN

SERVES FOR
4 PEOPLE

NUTRITION: calories 90.5, protein: 1.3g, carbs: 4g, fat: 7.7g

Parsley and Corn Salad

INGREDIENTS

- o   1 and 1/2 teaspoons balsamic vinegar
- o   2 tablespoons lime juice
- o   2 tablespoons olive oil
- o   A pinch of sea salt
- o   Black pepper to the taste
- o   4 cups corn
- o   black pepper
- o   1/2 cup parsley, chopped
- o   2 spring onions, chopped

DIRECTIONS:

1. In a salad bowl, combine the corn with the onions and the rest of the ingredients, toss, and serve cold.

PREPARATION
10 MIN

COOKING
0 MIN

SERVES FOR
4 PEOPLE

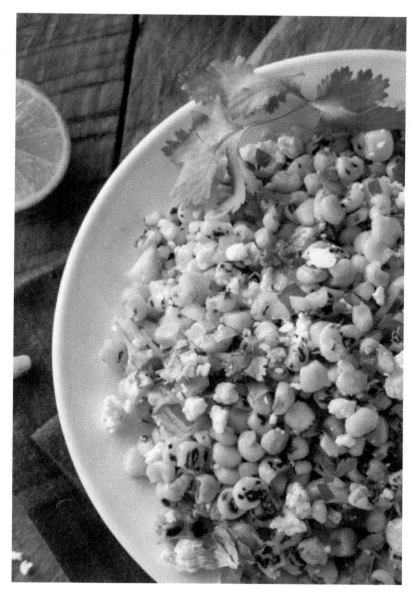

NUTRITION: Calories 121, Fat 9.5, Fiber 1.8, Carbs 4.1, Protein 1.9

Pear & brie salad

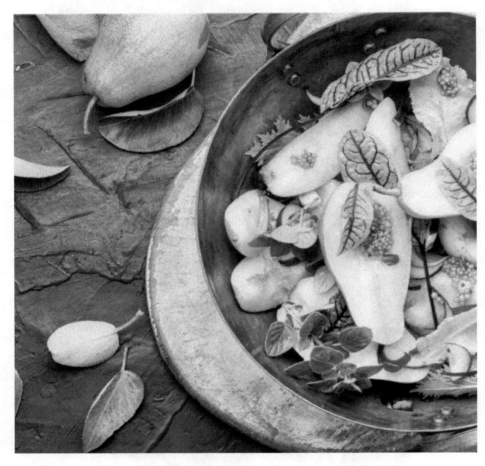

INGREDIENTS

- o 1/4 cucumber
- o /2 cup canned pears, juices drained
- o 1 cup arugula
- o 1/4 cup brie, chopped
- o 1/2 lemon
- o 1 tbsp olive oil

DIRECTIONS:

1. Peel and dice the cucumber.
2. Dice the pear.
3. Wash the arugula.
4. Combine salad in a serving bowl and crumble the brie over the top.
5. Whisk the olive oil and lemon juice together.
6. Drizzle over the salad.
7. Season with a little black pepper to taste and serve immediately.

PREPARATION
10 MIN

COOKING
0 MIN

SERVES FOR
4 PEOPLE

NUTRITION: calories 54, fat 7, fiber 5, carbs 15, protein 1

Kidney-friendly salad

INGREDIENTS

o 4 parsnips, peeled and sliced

o 1 tbsp extra virgin olive oil

o 1 tsp black pepper

o 1 tsp thyme

o 1 tsp chili flakes

DIRECTIONS:

1. Heat oven to 375°f/190°c/gas mark 5.

2. Grease a baking tray with the olive oil.

3. Add the parsnip slices in a thin layer.

4. Sprinkle over the thyme and chili slices and toss to coat.

5. Bake for 40-50 minutes

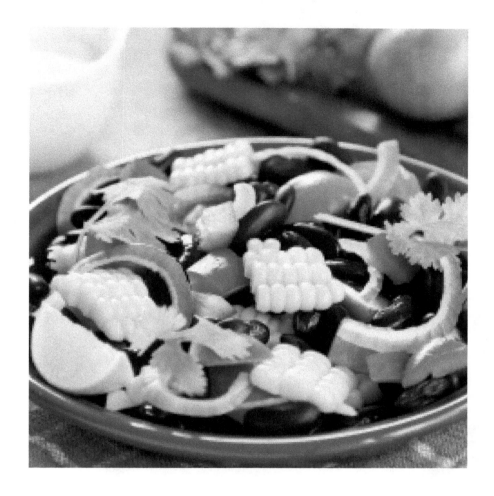

NUTRITION: calories 64, fat 4, fiber 1, carbs 5, protein 0

Beef Taco Salad

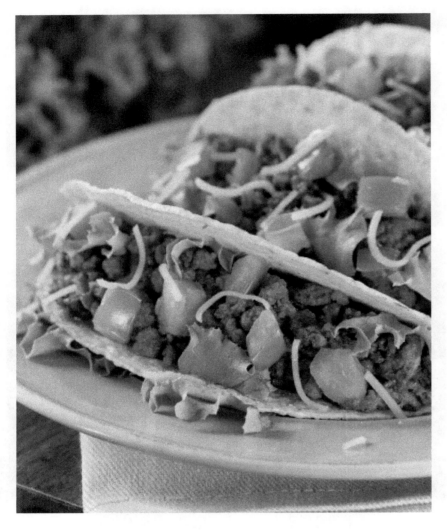

INGREDIENTS

- o 95 to 97% lean ground beef - 4.5 oz. when cooked (6.5 oz. - 3/4 leaner -lean)
- o Low-sodium taco seasoning mix (1.5 tsp. - condiment)
- o Water (2 tbsp.)
- o Lettuce - chopped (2 cups - greens)
- o Tomatoes (0.5 cup - greens)
- o 2% Reduced-fat Mexican Cheese (1 oz./0.25 cup - 1/4 of 1 lean)
- o Hidden Valley Light Ranch Dressing (2 tbsp. - healthy fat)

DIRECTION:

1. Prepare the veggies by chopping the lettuce and tomatoes; set them aside for now.

2. Warm a skillet to cook the beef. Drain the fat and toss back into the pan. Pour in the seasoning mix and water. Simmer for about five minutes.

3. Serve as desired with the meat over the bed of lettuce and tomatoes.

Sprinkle with Mexican cheese and dressing.

PREPARATION
10 MIN

COOKING
30 MIN

SERVES FOR
1 PEOPLE

NUTRITION: calories 160, fat 8, fiber 2, carbs 6, protein 3

Caprese Salad

INGREDIENTS

o Fresh mozzarella (4 oz. - 1 lean)

o 1 cup of greens Baby spinach

o 1 cup/180g – greens of Roma or heirloom tomatoes

o 0.25 cup of condiment of Fresh basil

o 1/8 tsp. of Black pepper & salt

o Walden Farms Balsamic Vinaigrette Dressing (2 tbsp. - condiment)

DIRECTIONS:

1. Slice the tomatoes and chop the basil. Cube the mozzarella.

2. Arrange the spinach greens on a plate and add the tomatoes, pepper, and salt.

3. Drizzle with the dressing and cheese with a sprinkling of fresh basil to serve.

Note: The mozzarella should contain 3-6 grams of fat per ounce.

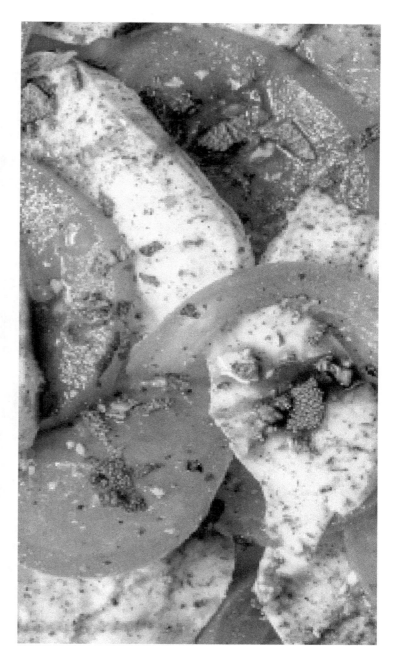

PREPARATION
10 MIN

COOKING
30 MIN

SERVES FOR
4 PEOPLE

NUTRITION: calories 90, fat 8, fiber 3, carbs 10, protein 2

Parsley Cheese Balls

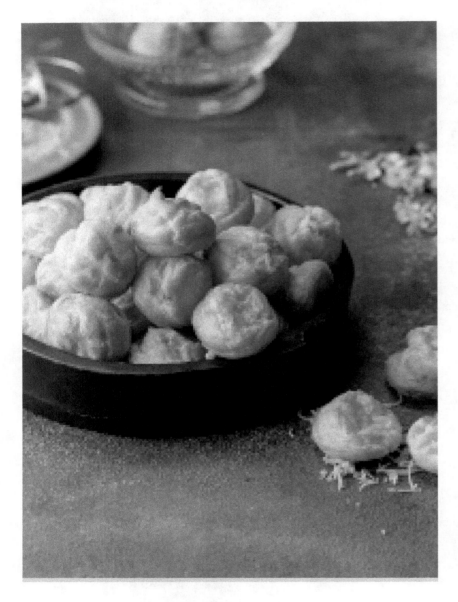

INGREDIENTS

o 1/3 cup Cheddar cheese, shredded

o 1 tablespoon dried dill

o 1 egg, beaten

o 1/2 teaspoon salt

o 2 tablespoons coconut flakes

o 3 tablespoons sunflower oil

DIRECTIONS

1. Mix up together shredded cheese with dried dill, salt, and coconut flakes.

2. Then add egg and stir carefully until homogenous.

3. After this make small balls from the cheese mixture.

4. Heat up sunflower oil in the skillet.

5. Place cheese balls in the hot oil and roast them for 10 seconds from each side.

6. Dry the cooked cheese balls with the help of a paper towel.

PREPARATION
10 MIN

COOKING
1 MIN

SERVES FOR
6 PEOPLE

NUTRITION: Calories 105, fat 10.4, fiber 0.2, carbs 0.7, protein 2.6

Chapter 11: Vegetables Recipes
Radish and Corn Salad

INGREDIENTS

- o 1 tablespoon lemon juice
- o black pepper
- o 1 jalapeno, chopped
- o 2 tablespoons olive oil
- o 1/4 teaspoon oregano, dried
- o A pinch of sea salt
- o 2 cups fresh corn
- o 6 radishes, sliced

DIRECTIONS

1. In a salad bowl, combine the corn with the radishes and the rest of the ingredients, toss, and serve cold.

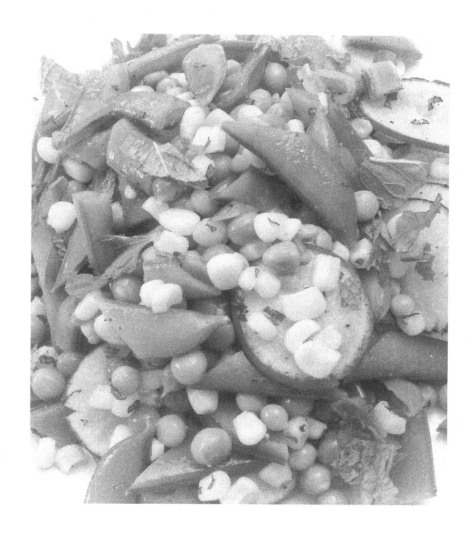

PREPARATION
10 MIN

COOKING
0 MIN

SERVES FOR
2 PEOPLE

NUTRITION: calories 134, fat 4.5, fiber 1.8, carbs 4.1, protein 1.9

Arugula and Corn Salad

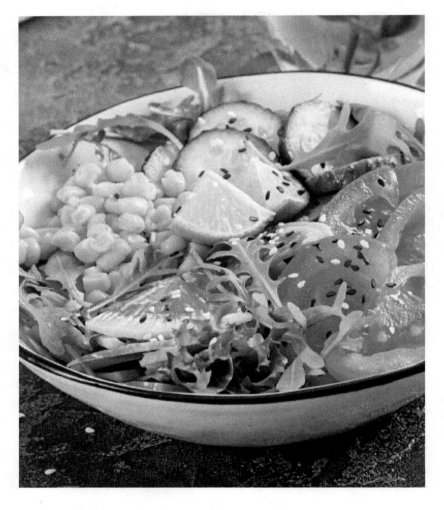

INGREDIENTS

o   1 red bell pepper, thinly sliced

o   2 cups corn

o   Juice of 1 lime

o   Salt

o   Pepper

o   Zest of 1 lime, grated

o   8 cups baby arugula

DIRECTIONS

1.   In a salad bowl, mix the corn with the arugula and the rest of the ingredients, toss and serve cold.

PREPARATION
10 MIN

COOKING
0 MIN

SERVES FOR
4 PEOPLE

NUTRITION: calories 172, fat 8.5, fiber 1.8, carbs 5.1, protein 1.4

Stir Fried Bok Choy

INGREDIENTS

- o 3 tablespoons coconut oil
- o 4 cloves of garlic, minced
- o 1 onion, chopped
- o 2 heads bok choy, rinsed and chopped
- o 2 teaspoons coconut aminos
- o Salt and pepper to taste
- o 2 tablespoons sesame oil
- o 2 tablespoons sesame seeds, toasted

DIRECTIONS

1. Heat the oil in a pot for 2 minutes.
2. Sauté the garlic and onions until fragrant, around 3 minutes.
3. Stir in the bok choy, coconut aminos, salt and pepper.
4. Cover pan and cook for 5 minutes.
5. Stir and continue cooking for another 3 minutes.
6. Drizzle with sesame oil and sesame seeds on top before serving.

PREPARATION
5 MIN

COOKING
13 MIN

SERVES FOR
4 PEOPLE

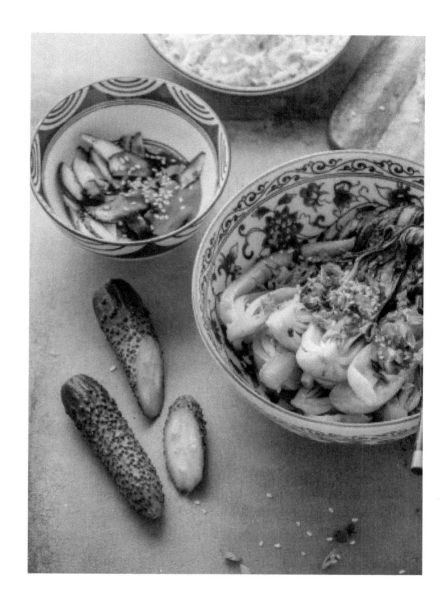

NUTRITION: calories: 358; carbs: 5.2g; protein: 21.5g; fat: 28.4g

Summer Veggies Pot

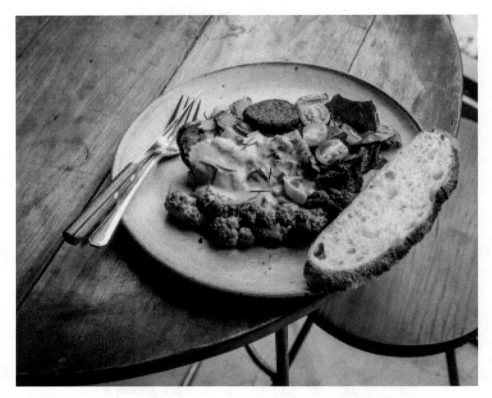

PREPARATION
10 MIN

COOKING
7 MIN

SERVES FOR
6 PEOPLE

INGREDIENTS

o 2 cups okra, sliced

o 1 cup grape tomatoes

o 1 cup mushroom, sliced

o 1 1/2 cups onion, sliced

o 2 cups bell pepper, sliced

o 2 1/2 cups zucchini, sliced

o 2 tablespoons basil, chopped

o 1 tablespoon thyme, chopped

o 1/2 cups balsamic vinegar

o 1/2 cups olive oil

o Salt and pepper

DIRECTIONS

1. Place all ingredients in the Instant Pot.

2. Stir the contents and close the lid.

3. Close the lid and press the Manual button.

4. Adjust the Cooking Time to 7 minutes.

5. Do quick pressure release.

6. Once cooled, evenly divide into serving size, keep in your preferred container, and refrigerate until ready to eat.

NUTRITION: calories per serving: 233; carbs: 7g; protein: 3g; fat:

Stir Fried Asparagus and Bell Pepper

PREPARATION
10 MIN

COOKING
10 MIN

SERVES FOR
6 PEOPLE

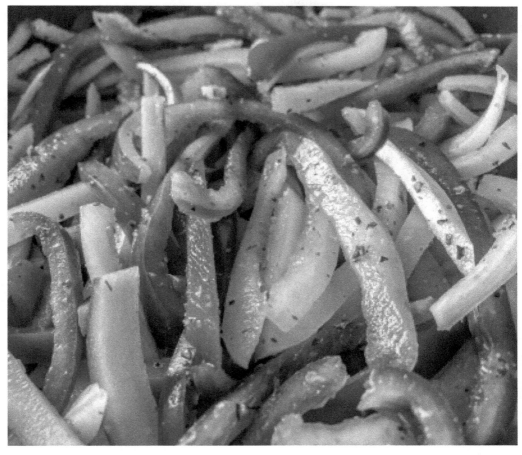

INGREDIENTS

o   1 tablespoon olive oil

o   4 cloves of garlic, minced

o   1-pound fresh asparagus spears, trimmed

o   2 large red bell peppers, seeded and julienned

o   1/2 teaspoon thyme

o   5 tablespoons water

o   1/2 tsp salt

o   1/2 tsp pepper or more to taste

DIRECTIONS

1.   Place a nonstick saucepan on high fire and heat pan for a minute.

2.   Add oil and heat for 2 minutes.

3.   Stir in garlic and sauté for a minute.

4.   Add remaining ingredients and stir fry until soft and tender, around 6 minutes.

5.   Turn off fire, let veggies rest while the pan is covered for 5 minutes.

Serve and enjoy.

NUTRITION: calories 44, fat 2, fiber 5, carbs 15, protein 2

Stir Fried Kale

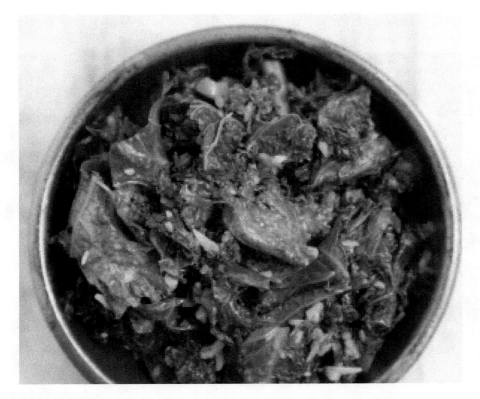

PREPARATION
10 MIN

COOKING
10 MIN

SERVES FOR
6 PEOPLE

INGREDIENTS

o   1 tablespoon coconut oil

o   2 cloves of garlic, minced

o   1 onion, chopped

o   2 teaspoons crushed red pepper flakes

o   4 cups kale, chopped

o   2 tbsp water

o   Salt and pepper to taste

DIRECTIONS:

1.   Place a nonstick saucepan on high fire and heat pan for a minute.

2.   Add oil and heat for 2 minutes.

3.   Stir in garlic and sauté for a minute. Add onions and stir fry for another minute.

4.   Add remaining ingredients and stir fry until soft and tender, around 4 minutes.

5.   Turn off fire, let veggies rest while the pan is covered for 3 minutes.

Serve and enjoy.

NUTRITION: calories 37, fat 2, fiber 1, carbs 5, protein 1

Sweet Potato Puree

PREPARATION
10 MIN

COOKING
15 MIN

SERVES FOR
6 PEOPLE

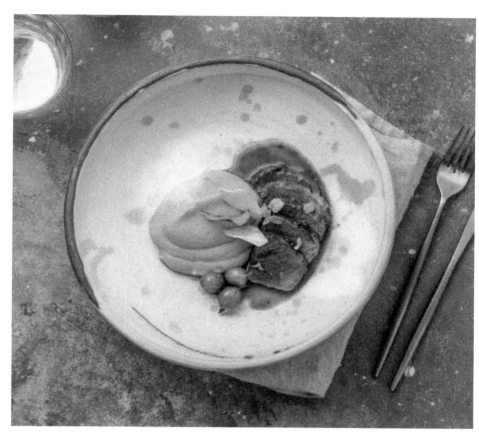

INGREDIENTS

o   2 pounds sweet potatoes, peeled

o   1 1/2 cups water

o   5 Medjool dates, pitted and chopped

DIRECTIONS

1.   Place water and potatoes in a pot.

2.   Close the lid and allow to boil for 15 minutes until the potatoes are soft.

3.   Drain the potatoes and place in a food processor together with the dates.

4.   Pulse until smooth.

Serve and enjoy.

NUTRITION: calories 174, fat 1, fiber 5, carbs 45, protein 3

Curried Okra

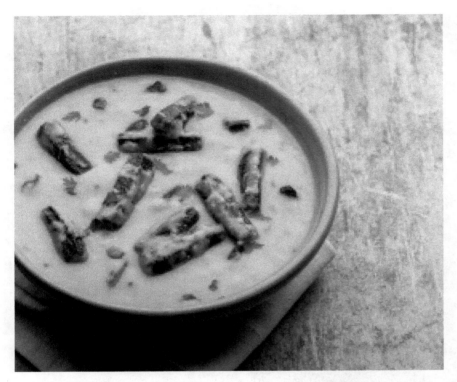

PREPARATION
10 MIN

COOKING
12 MIN

SERVES FOR
4 PEOPLE

INGREDIENTS

o 1 lb. small to medium okra pods, trimmed

o 1/4 tsp curry powder

o 1/2 tsp kosher salt

o 1 tsp finely chopped serrano chile

o 1 tsp ground coriander

o 1 tbsp canola oil

o 3/4 tsp brown mustard seeds

DIRECTIONS

1. On medium-high fire, place a large and heavy skillet and cook mustard seeds until fragrant, around 30 seconds.

2. Add canola oil. Add okra, curry powder, salt, chile, and coriander. Sauté for a minute while stirring every once in a while.

3. Cover and cook low fire for at least 8 minutes. Stir occasionally.

4. Uncover, increase the fire to medium-high and cook until okra is lightly browned, around 2 minutes more.

Serve and enjoy.

NUTRITION: calories 74, fat 6, fiber 3, carbs 5, protein 2

Zucchini Pasta with Mango-Kiwi Sauce

PREPARATION
10 MIN

COOKING
0 MIN

SERVES FOR
2 PEOPLE

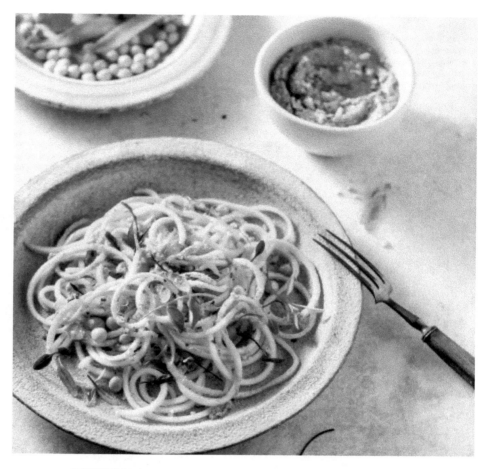

INGREDIENTS

- o 1 tsp dried herbs – optional
- o 1/2 Cup Raw Kale leaves, shredded
- o 2 small dried figs
- o 3 medjool dates
- o 4 medium kiwis
- o 2 big mangos, peeled and seed discarded
- o 2 cup zucchini, spiralized
- o 1/4 cup roasted cashew

DIRECTIONS

1. On a salad bowl, place kale then topped with zucchini noodles, and sprinkle with dried herbs. Set aside.

2. In a food processor, grind to a powder the cashews. Add figs, dates, kiwis, and mangoes then puree to a smooth consistency.

3. Pour over zucchini pasta, serve and enjoy.

NUTRITION: calories 224, fat 12, fiber 5, carbs 15, protein 5

Herb Flavored Potato Soup

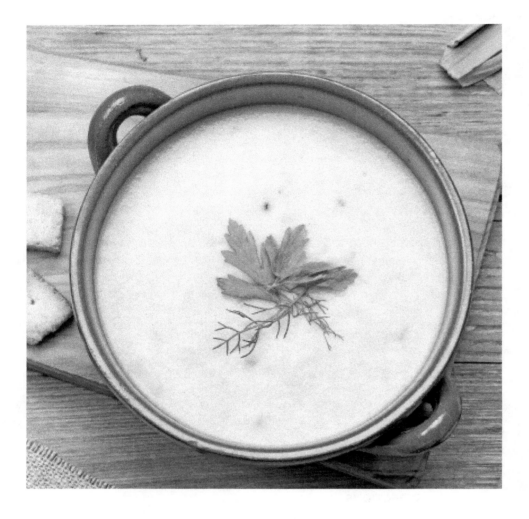

PREPARATION
10 MIN

COOKING
12 MIN

SERVES FOR
4 PEOPLE

INGREDIENTS

o   3 medium potatoes

o   2 tbsp ginger, minced

o   Salt and pepper

o   3 cups vegetable broth

o   2 tbsp rosemary, chopped

DIRECTIONS:

1.   Put all the ingredients in the instant pot cooker and lock the lid. Cook with Soup setting for 15 minutes and then let the pressure release naturally.

2.   Open the lid of the instant pot and simmer the soup for another 5 minutes. Use a hand blender to make the soup smooth.

3.   Serve hot by seasoning with some more pepper and salt.

NUTRITION: calories 74, fat 6, fiber 3, carbs 5, protein 2

Greek Cauliflower Rice

PREPARATION
10 MIN

COOKING
12 MIN

SERVES FOR
2 PEOPLE

INGREDIENTS

1/2 cup cauliflower rice

1 tbsp pecans, toasted and chopped

1/2 tbsp fresh lime juice

1 1/3 cup vegetable stock

3 oz spinach, chopped

1/4 cup water

1 tbsp olive oil

1/2 small onion, chopped

1/2 tsp garlic, minced

1/4 cup grape tomatoes, halved

2 tbsp feta cheese, crumbled

Salt

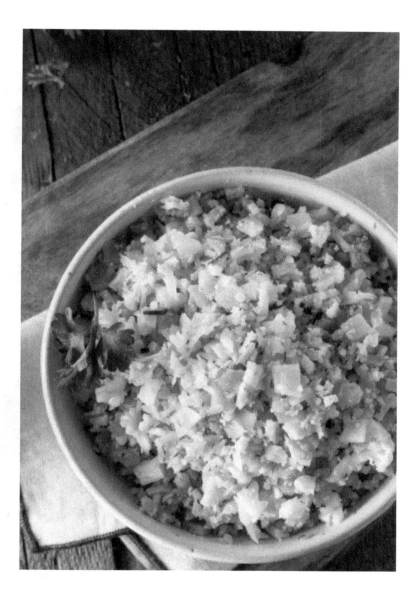

DIRECTIONS

1. Add oil into the inner pot of instant pot and set the pot on sauté mode.

2. Add garlic and onion and sauté for 5 minutes.

3. Add cauliflower rice, water, and stock and stir well.

4. Seal pot with lid and cook on high for 4 minutes.

5. Once done, release pressure using quick release. Remove lid.

6. Add spinach and tomatoes and cook on sauté mode for 3 minutes.

7. Add remaining ingredients and stir well and serve.

NUTRITION: calories 174, fat 16, fiber 3, carbs 9, protein 5

Chapter 12: Fish and Seafood Recipes

Sardine Fish Cakes

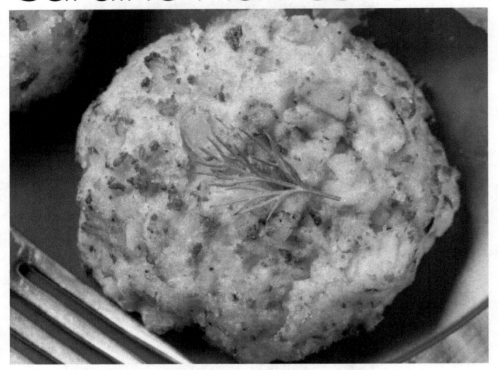

PREPARATION
10 MIN

COOKING
10 MIN

SERVES FOR
4 PEOPLE

INGREDIENTS

o   11 oz sardines, canned, drained

o   1/3 cup shallot, chopped

o   1 teaspoon chili flakes

o   1/2 teaspoon salt

o   2 tablespoon wheat flour, whole grain

o   1 egg, beaten

o   1 tablespoon chives, chopped

o   1 teaspoon olive oil

o   1 teaspoon butter

DIRECTIONS

1.   Put the butter in the skillet and melt it.

2.   Add shallot and cook it until translucent.

3.   After this, transfer the shallot in the mixing bowl.

4.   Add sardines, chili flakes, salt, flour, egg, chives, and mix up until smooth with the help of the fork.

5.   Make the medium size cakes and place them in the skillet.

6.   Add olive oil.

7.   Roast the fish cakes for 3 minutes from each side over the medium heat.

8.   Dry the cooked fish cakes with a paper towel if needed and transfer in the serving plates.

NUTRITION: calories 221, fat 12.2, fiber 0.1, carbs 5.4, protein 21.3

Cajun Catfish

PREPARATION
10 MIN

COOKING
10 MIN

SERVES FOR
4 PEOPLE

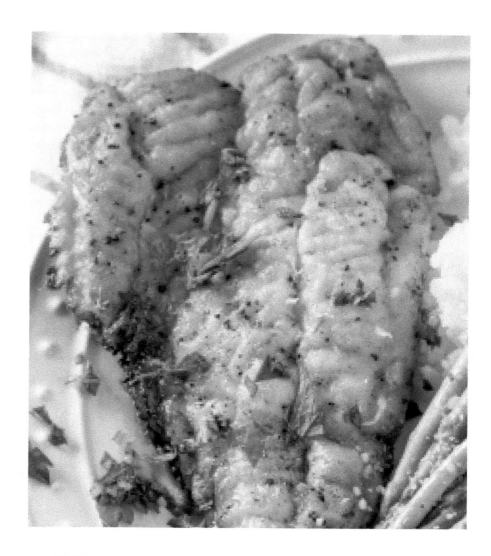

INGREDIENTS

o   16 oz catfish steaks (4 oz each fish steak)

o   1 tablespoon Cajun spices

o   1 egg, beaten

o   1 tablespoon sunflower oil

DIRECTIONS:

1. Pour sunflower oil in the skillet and preheat it until shimmering.

2. Meanwhile, dip every catfish steak in the beaten egg and coat it in Cajun spices.

3. Place the fish steaks in the hot oil and roast them for 4 minutes from each side.

4. The cooked catfish steaks should have a light brown crust.

NUTRITION: calories 263, fat 16.7, fiber 0, carbs 0.1, protein 26.3

Seabass with Red Peppers

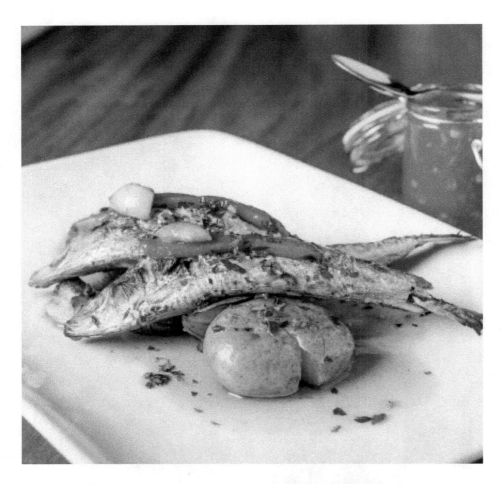

PREPARATION
10 MIN

COOKING
40 MIN

SERVES FOR
4 PEOPLE

INGREDIENTS

o 2 red peppers, trimmed

o 11 oz Gennaro/seabass, trimmed

o 1 teaspoon salt

o 1/2 teaspoon ground black pepper

o 2 tablespoons butter

o 1 lemon

DIRECTIONS

1. Remove the seeds from red peppers and cut them on the wedges.

2. Then line the baking tray with parchment and arrange red peppers in a layer.

3. Rub Gennaro/seabass with ground black pepper and salt and place it on the peppers.

4. Then add butter.

5. Cut the lemon on the halves and squeeze the juice over the fish.

6. Bake the fish for 40 minutes at 350F.

NUTRITION: calories 148, fat 10.3, fiber 1.2, carbs 7.3, protein 8.5

Salmon Fillet

PREPARATION
5 MIN

COOKING
25 MIN

SERVES FOR
1 PEOPLE

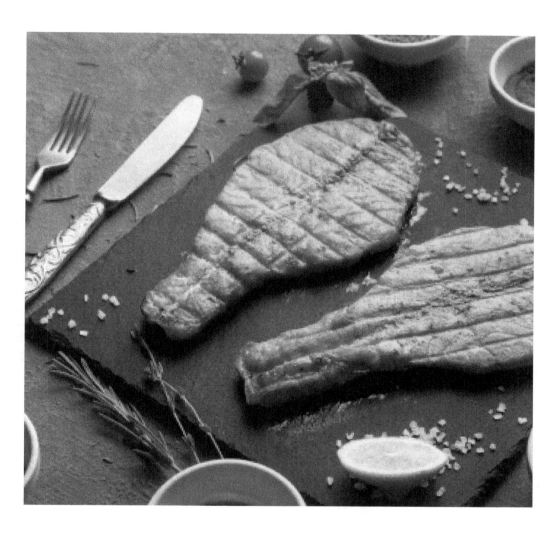

INGREDIENTS

o   4 oz salmon fillet

o   1/2 teaspoon salt

o   1 teaspoon sesame oil

o   1/2 teaspoon sage

DIRECTIONS

1.   Rub the fillet with salt and sage.

2.   Place the fish in the tray and sprinkle it with sesame oil.

3.   Cook the fish for 25 minutes at 365F.

4.   Flip the fish carefully onto another side after 12 minutes of cooking.

NUTRITION: calories 191, fat 11.6, fiber 0.1, carbs 0.2, protein 22

Mango Tilapia Fillets

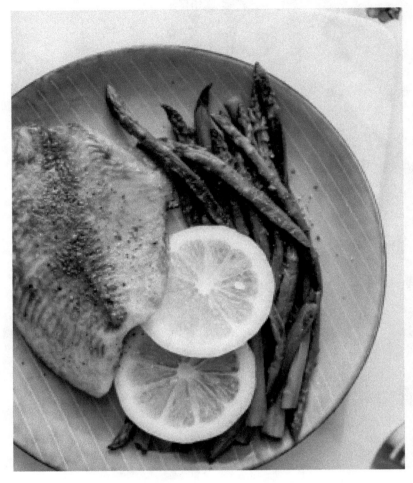

INGREDIENTS

o   1/4 cup coconut flakes

o   5 oz mango, peeled

o   1/3 cup shallot, chopped

o   1 teaspoon ground turmeric

o   1 cup of water

o   1 bay leaf

o   12 oz tilapia fillets

o   1 chili pepper, chopped

o   1 tablespoon coconut oil

o   1/2 teaspoon salt

o   1 teaspoon paprika

DIRECTIONS

1. Blend coconut flakes, mango, shallot, ground turmeric, and water.

2. After this, melt coconut oil in the saucepan.

3. Sprinkle the tilapia fillets with salt and paprika.

4. Then place them in the hot coconut oil and roast for 1 minute from each side.

5. Add chili pepper, bay leaf, and blended mango mixture.

6. Close the lid and cook the fish for 10 minutes over the medium heat.

PREPARATION
10 MIN

COOKING
15 MIN

SERVES FOR
4 PEOPLE

NUTRITION: calories 153, fat 6.1, fiber 1.5, carbs 9.3, protein 16.8

Seafood Gratin

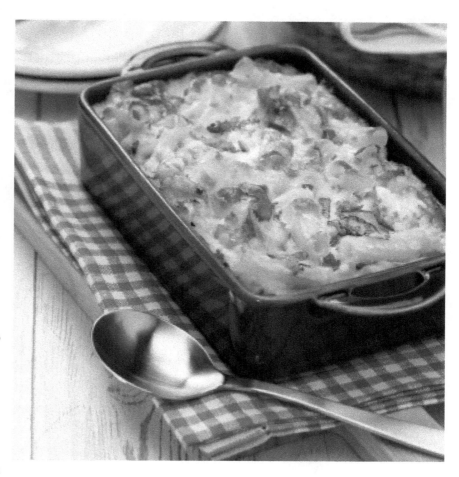

INGREDIENTS

- 3 Russet potatoes, sliced
- 1/2 cup onion, chopped
- 1/2 cup milk
- 1 egg, beaten
- 3 tablespoon wheat flour, whole grain
- 1 cup shrimps, peeled
- 1/2 cup Mozzarella cheese, shredded
- 1/4 cup Cheddar cheese, shredded
- 1 teaspoon olive oil
- 1 cup water, for cooking

DIRECTIONS

1. Pour water into the pan and bring it to a boil.
2. Add sliced potatoes to the hot water and boil it for 3 minutes.
3. Then remove potatoes from water.
4. Mix up together beaten egg, milk, chopped onion, flour, and Cheddar cheese.
5. Preheat the mixture until the cheese is melted.
6. Then place the potatoes in the gratin mold in one layer.
7. Add the layer of shrimps.
8. Pour Cheddar cheese mixture over shrimps and top the gratin with Mozzarella cheese.
9. Cover the gratin with foil and secure the edges.
10. Bake gratin for 35 minutes at 355F.

PREPARATION
15 MIN

COOKING
40 MIN

SERVES FOR
5 PEOPLE

NUTRITION: calories 205, fat 5.3, fiber 3.5, carbs 26.2, protein 14.1

Teriyaki Tuna

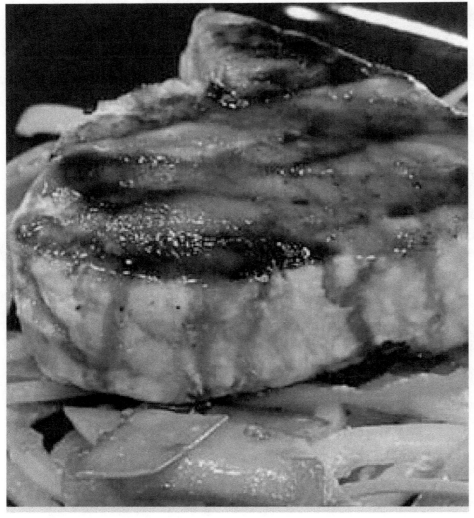

INGREDIENTS

o 3 tuna fillets

o 3 teaspoons teriyaki sauce

o 1/2 teaspoon minced garlic

o 1 teaspoon olive oil

DIRECTIONS

1. Whisk together teriyaki sauce, minced garlic, and olive oil.

2. Brush every tuna fillet with teriyaki mixture.

3. Preheat grill to 390F.

4. Grill the fish for 3 minutes from each side.

PREPARATION
10 MIN

COOKING
6 MIN

SERVES FOR
3 PEOPLE

NUTRITION: calories 382, fat 32.6, fiber 0, carbs 1.1, protein 21.4

Tandoori Salmon Skewers

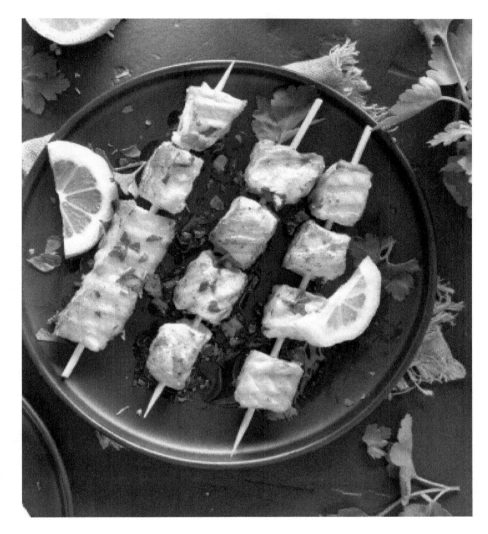

INGREDIENTS

o   1.5-pound salmon fillet

o   1/2 cup Plain yogurt

o   1 teaspoon paprika

o   1 teaspoon turmeric

o   1 teaspoon red pepper

o   1 teaspoon salt

o   1 teaspoon dried cilantro

o   1 teaspoon sunflower oil

o   1/2 teaspoon ground nutmeg

DIRECTIONS

1. For the marinade: mix up together Plain yogurt, paprika, turmeric red pepper, salt, and ground nutmeg.

2. Chop the salmon fillet roughly and put it in the yogurt mixture.

3. Mix up well and marinate for 25 minutes.

4. Then skew the fish on the skewers.

5. Sprinkle the skewers with sunflower oil and place them in the tray.

6. Bake the salmon skewers for 15 minutes at 375F.

PREPARATION
30 MIN

COOKING
15 MIN

SERVES FOR
5 PEOPLE

NUTRITION: calories 217, fat 9.9, fiber 0.6, carbs 4.2, protein 28.1

Tuna and Vegetable Kebabs

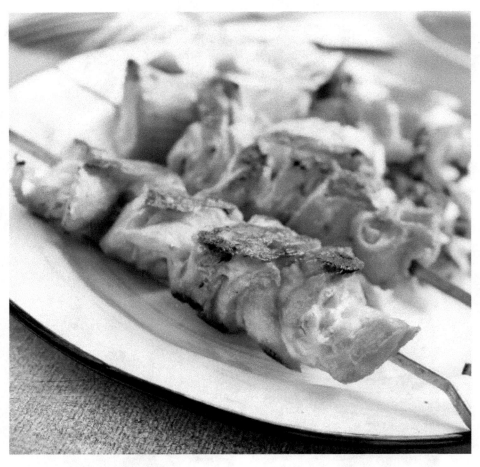

INGREDIENTS

o 1/2 teaspoon rosemary

o 1 pound 1 1/4 -inch-thick tuna, cut into bite-sized cubes

o 1 onion, cut into wedges

o 1 cup grape tomatoes

o 2 tablespoons soy sauce

o 1/2 teaspoon thyme

o Salt and crushed black peppercorns

o 1 zucchini, diced

o 2 tablespoons olive oil

DIRECTIONS

1. Firstly, preheat your grill on high. Season tuna cubes and vegetables with peppercorns, salt, rosemary, and thyme. After that, drizzle with the oil and soy sauce.

2. Succeeding the above, alternate seasoned tuna cubes, zucchini, onion, and tomatoes on each of 8 metal skewers.

3. Now, grill 5 minutes for medium-rare, turning frequently. Bon appetite!

PREPARATION
30 MIN

COOKING
15 MIN

SERVES FOR
5 PEOPLE

NUTRITION: calories 74, fat 6, fiber 3, carbs 5, protein 2

Mackerel Steak Casserole

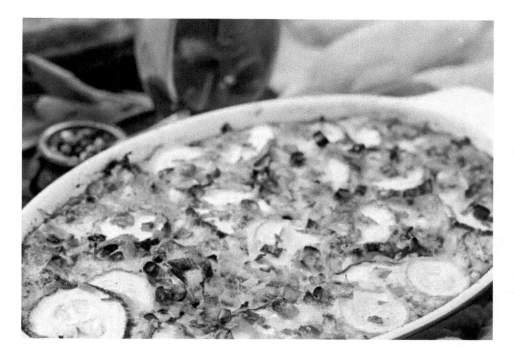

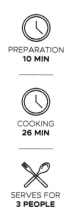

PREPARATION
10 MIN

COOKING
26 MIN

SERVES FOR
3 PEOPLE

INGREDIENTS

o   2 cloves garlic, thinly sliced

o   Salt and black pepper, to your liking

o   1 tablespoon Old Bay seasoning

o   1 cup mozzarella, shredded

o   1/2 stick butter

o   1 pound mackerel steaks

o   1/2 cup fresh chives, chopped

o   1/4 cup clam juice

o   2 onions, thinly sliced

o   3 tomatoes, thinly sliced

DIRECTIONS

1.   Firstly, preheat your oven to 4500F.

2.   Dissolve the butter in a pan that is previously preheated over a normal flame. Heat the garlic and onions until they are tender.

3.   Include clam juice and tomatoes and cook for 4 minutes more. Put this vegetable mixture into a casserole dish.

4.   Then, Lay the fish steaks on top of the vegetable layer. Spray with seasonings. Close with foil and roast for about 10 minutes until the fish is opaque in the center.

5.   Now, top with shredded cheese and bake for another 5 minutes. Enjoy warm garnished with fresh chopped chives.

NUTRITION: calories 304, fat 6, fiber 3, carbs 6, protein 33

Smoky Cholula Seafood Dip

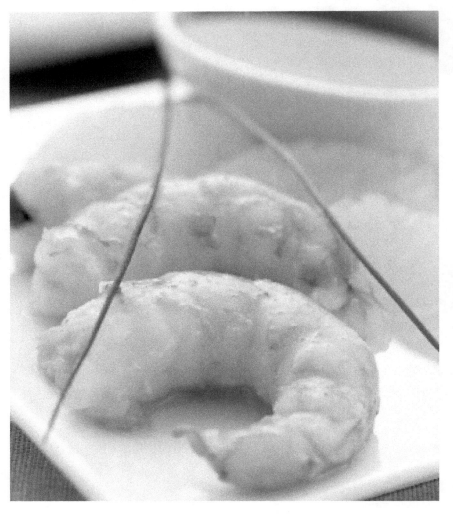

INGREDIENTS

o Sea salt and ground black pepper, to taste

o 1/2 cup mayonnaise

o 1 tablespoon Cholula

o 12 ounces seafood, canned and drained

o 1/2 teaspoon dried dill weed

o 2 cloves garlic, finely minced

o 1/4 teaspoon white pepper

o A few drops of liquid smoke

o 1 teaspoon smoked paprika

DIRECTIONS

1. In a mixing container, gently stir garlic, mayo, and canned seafood.

2. Include the remaining ingredients and stir with a wide spatula until everything is well merged.

3. Close the lid and place it in your refrigerator until it is thoroughly chilled. Enjoy well-chilled with fresh or pickled veggies.

PREPARATION
10 MIN

COOKING
6 MIN

SERVES FOR
3 PEOPLE

NUTRITION: calories 104, fat 6, fiber 3, carbs 5, protein 9

Smoked Creamy Fish Fat Bombs

INGREDIENTS

o   1/4 cup of mayonnaise

o   1 cup cream cheese

o   1 tbsp of mustard

o   1 filet smoked fish, boneless, crumbled

o   2 Tbsp grated cheese

o   1 tsp fresh parsley, chopped

DIRECTIONS

1. Combine all ingredients and beat in a food processor.

2. Make 6 balls and place them on a lined pan with parchment paper.

3. Refrigerate for 3 hours.

4. Serve cold.

PREPARATION
10 MIN

COOKING
6 MIN

SERVES FOR
3 PEOPLE

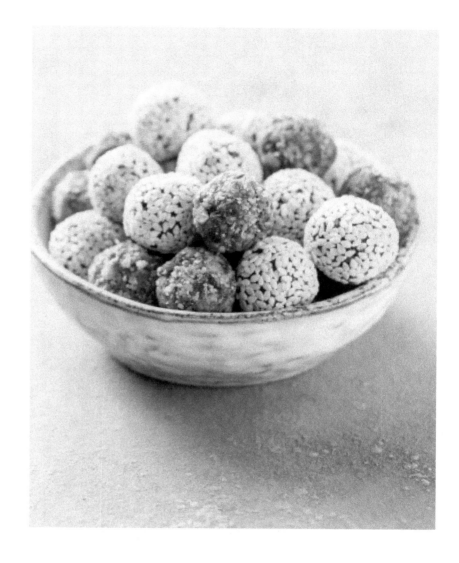

NUTRITION: calories 174, fat 16, fiber 3, carbs 9, protein 5

Indian Fish Fry

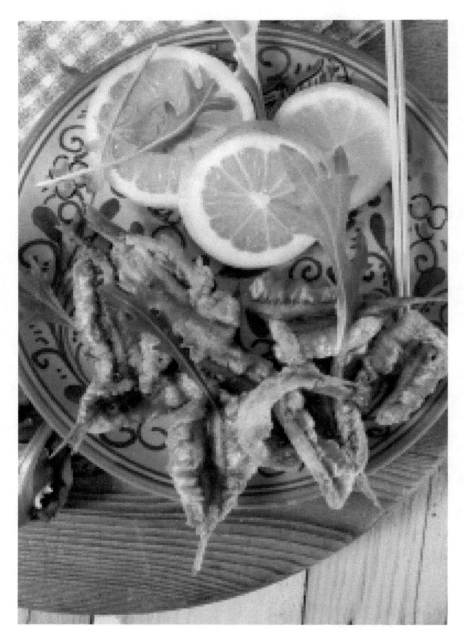

INGREDIENTS

o 3 carp fillets

o 1/2 teaspoon garam masala

o 3 tablespoons full-fat coconut milk

o 1 egg

o 2 tablespoons olive oil

DIRECTIONS

1. Pat the fish fillets dry with pepper towels. Toss fish fillets with garam masala along with sea salt and black pepper.

2. In a mixing dish, beat the coconut milk and egg until pale and frothy. Dip the fillets into the milk/egg mixture.

3. Heat olive oil in a frying pan over medium-high heat. Fry the fish fillets until they begin to flake when tested with a fork.

4. Serve with curry leaves if desired and enjoy!

PREPARATION
10 MIN

COOKING
6 MIN

SERVES FOR
3 PEOPLE

NUTRITION: calories 444, fat 16, fiber 3, carbs 35, protein 23

Tilapia and Shrimp Soup

INGREDIENTS

- 1 cup celery, chopped
- 2 cups cauliflower, grated
- 2 cups tomato sauce with onion and garlic
- 1 pound tilapia, skinless and chopped into small chunks
- 1/2 pound medium shrimp, deveined

DIRECTIONS

1. Melt 2 tablespoons of butter in a soup pot over medium-high flame. Once hot, cook celery and cauliflower for 4 to 5 minutes or until tender.

2. Add in tomato sauce along with 4 cups of chicken broth and bring to a boil. Now, turn the heat to medium-low.

3. Stir in the tilapia and continue to cook, partially covered, for about 10 minutes. Stir in the shrimp and continue to simmer for 3 to 4 minutes or until shrimp is pink.

4. Ladle into soup bowls and serve hot!

PREPARATION
10 MIN

COOKING
26 MIN

SERVES FOR
3 PEOPLE

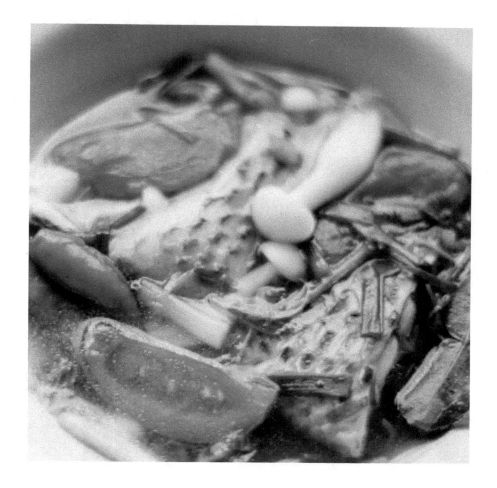

NUTRITION: calories 224, fat 6, fiber 3, carbs 5, protein 26

Chapter 13: Meat and Poultry Recipes

Roasted Spatchcock Chicken

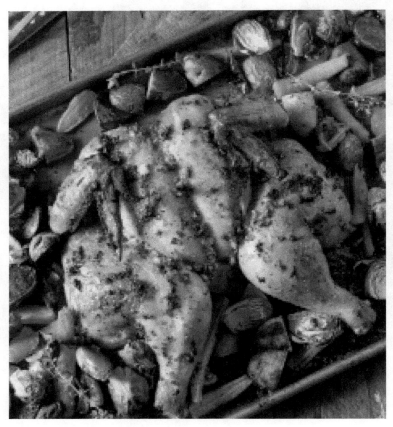

INGREDIENTS

- o 1 (4-pound) whole chicken
- o 1 (1-inch) piece fresh ginger, sliced
- o 4 garlic cloves, chopped
- o 1 small bunch of fresh thyme
- o Pinch of cayenne
- o Salt and freshly ground black pepper, to taste
- o 1/4 cup fresh lemon juice
- o 3 tablespoons extra virgin olive oil

DIRECTIONS

1. Arrange chicken, breast side down onto a large cutting board.
2. With a kitchen shear, begin with thigh and cut along 1 side of the backbone and turn chicken around.
3. Now, cut along sleep issues and discard the backbone.
4. Change the inside and open it like a book.
5. Flatten the backbone firmly to flatten.
6. In a food processor, add all ingredients except chicken and pulse till smooth.
7. In a big baking dish, add the marinade mixture.
8. Add chicken and coat with marinade generously.
9. With a plastic wrap, cover the baking dish and refrigerate to marinate for overnight.
10. Preheat the oven to 450 degrees F. Arrange a rack in a very roasting pan.
11. Remove the chicken from the refrigerator and make it onto a rack over a roasting pan, skin side down.
12. Roast for about 50 minutes, turning once in the middle way.

PREPARATION
10 MIN

COOKING
50 MIN

SERVES FOR
5 PEOPLE

NUTRITION: calories 374, fat 16, fiber 4, carbs 29, protein 45

Prosciutto Wrapped Turkey

INGREDIENTS

- o 2 pounds marinated turkey breasts
- o 1 1/2 tablespoons of coconut butter, room temperature
- o 1/2 teaspoon of chili powder
- o 1 teaspoon of cayenne pepper
- o 1 sprig finely chopped fresh thyme
- o 2 sprigs finely chopped rosemary
- o 2 tablespoons of Cabernet Sauvignon
- o 1 teaspoon of sea salt
- o 1/2 teaspoon of freshly ground black pepper
- o 1 teaspoon of finely minced garlic
- o 10 strips prosciutto

DIRECTIONS

1. Chop the turkey into 10 slices of the same size.

2. In a skillet, melt the coconut butter over medium heat. Cook the turkey breasts on both sides for 2 – 3 minutes each side.

3. Sprinkle the chili powder, cayenne pepper, thyme, rosemary, salt, pepper and garlic. Drizzle a little wine over the turkey. Wrap each slice of turkey with a prosciutto strip.

4. Put your oven on at 4500F. Place the turkey and prosciutto in a roasting pan and cook for 25 minutes.

5. Garnish with fresh cilantro.

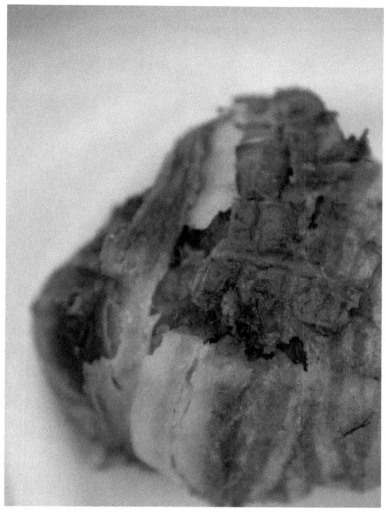

PREPARATION
10 MIN

COOKING
40 MIN

SERVES FOR
4 PEOPLE

NUTRITION: calories 274, fat 16, fiber 3, carbs 7, protein 40

Oven Baked Creamy Chicken Thighs

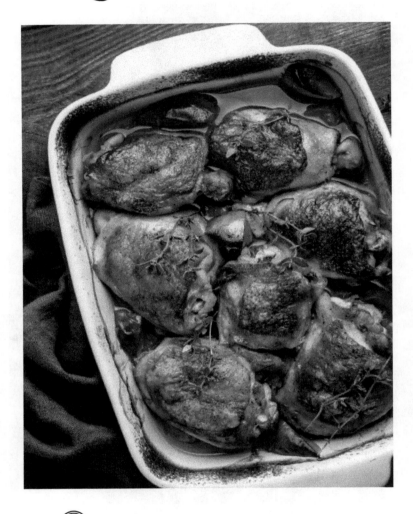

INGREDIENTS

o   3/4 cup mayonnaise

o   1/4 cup yellow mustard

o   1/2 cup Parmesan cheese freshly grated

o   1 tsp Italian seasoning

o   1/4 tsp of coriander

o   1/4 tsp of marjoram

o   2 lbs. chicken thighs (boneless and skinless)

o   1/2 tsp salt and ground black pepper

DIRECTIONS

1.   Preheat oven to 400 F/200 C.

2.   Oil one 8-inch square baking dish.

3.   In a bowl combine the mayonnaise, mustard, Parmesan cheese, coriander, marjoram, and Italian seasoning.

4.   Season generously chicken thigh with salt and pepper and place in a prepared baking dish.

5.   Spread with mayo-mustard sauce and bake for 35 - 40 minutes. Serve warm.

PREPARATION
10 MIN

COOKING
40 MIN

SERVES FOR
6 PEOPLE

NUTRITION: calories 174, fat 16, fiber 3, carbs 9, protein 5

Chicken and Romano Cheese

INGREDIENTS

o 1/2 pound chicken fillets

o 1 egg, whisked

o 3 ounces Romano cheese, grated

o 2 ounces pork rinds, crushed

o 1 large-sized Roma tomato, pureed

DIRECTIONS

1. In a shallow dish, place the whisked egg.

2. In the second shallow dish, mix Romano cheese and crushed pork rinds; season with salt, black pepper, cayenne pepper, and dried parsley.

3. Dip the chicken fillets into the egg mixture; then, roll the chicken over the breading mixture until well coated.

4. In a frying pan, heat 2 tablespoons of olive oil over medium-high heat. Once hot, fry the chicken fillets for about 3 minutes per side.

5. Place the chicken in a lightly greased baking pan. Spread pureed tomato over the top. Bake for a further 3 minutes.

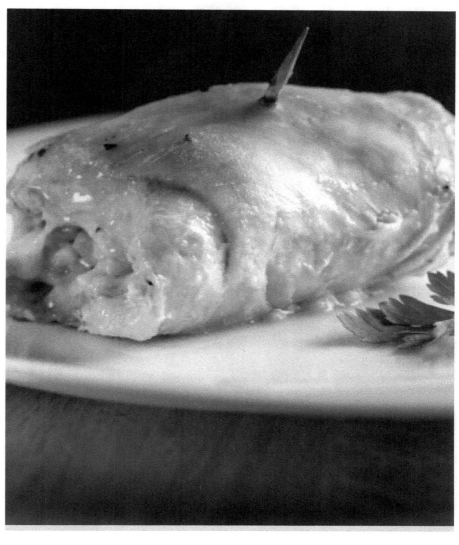

PREPARATION
10 MIN

COOKING
40 MIN

SERVES FOR
4 PEOPLE

NUTRITION: calories 374, fat 26, fiber 3, carbs 29, protein 22

Indian Chicken Masala

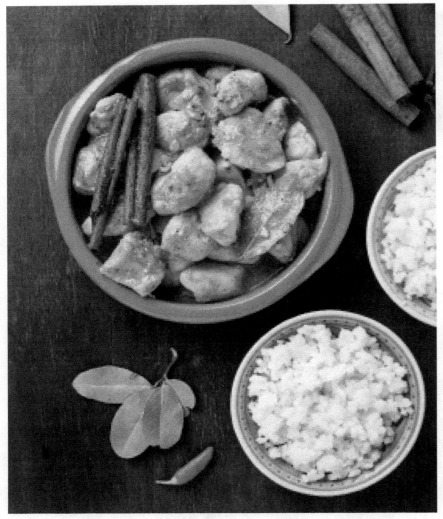

INGREDIENTS

o 1 1/2 pounds of chicken breasts, cut into bite-sized pieces

o 1 teaspoon of garam masala

o 10 ounces of tomato puree

o 1/2 cup of heavy cream

o 1 onion, chopped

DIRECTIONS

1. Spritz a saucepan with a nonstick cooking spray and preheat over medium-high heat. Now, sear the chicken breasts until nicely browned on both sides.

2. Remove the chicken to the sides of the saucepan and sauté the onions for about 3 minutes or until translucent and tender.

3. Stir in the garam masala and tomato puree. Cook for 9 to 10 minutes until the sauce is reduced by two-thirds.

4. Add in the heavy cream and stir for about 12 minutes or until thoroughly heated.

PREPARATION
10 MIN

COOKING
40 MIN

SERVES FOR
4 PEOPLE

NUTRITION: calories 320, fat 26, fiber 2, carbs 9, protein 24

Gourmet Italian Turkey Fillets

INGREDIENTS

o   2 eggs

o   1 cup of sour cream

o   1 teaspoon of Italian seasoning blend

o   1/2 cup of grated parmesan cheese

o   2 pounds of turkey fillets

DIRECTIONS

1. Beat the eggs until frothy and light. Add in the sour cream and continue whisking until pale and well mixed.

2. In another bowl, mix the Italian seasoning blend and parmesan cheese; mix to combine well.

3. Dip the turkey fillets into the egg mixture; then, coat them with the parmesan mixture.

4. Fry turkey fillets in the greased sauté pan until golden brown and cooked through.

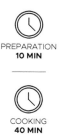

PREPARATION
10 MIN

COOKING
40 MIN

SERVES FOR
4 PEOPLE

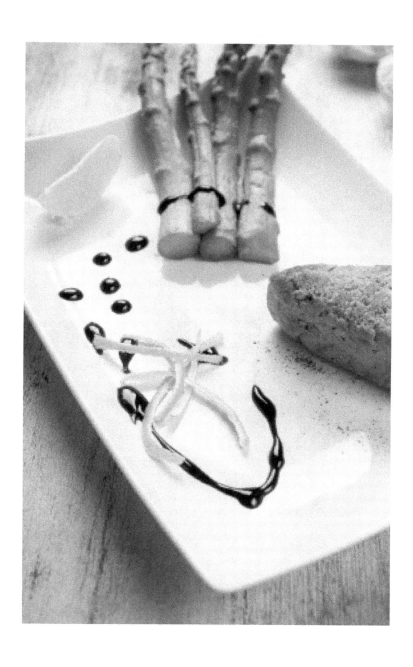

NUTRITION: calories 334, fat 6, fiber 1, carbs 21, protein 35

Mediterranean Chicken with Thyme and Olives

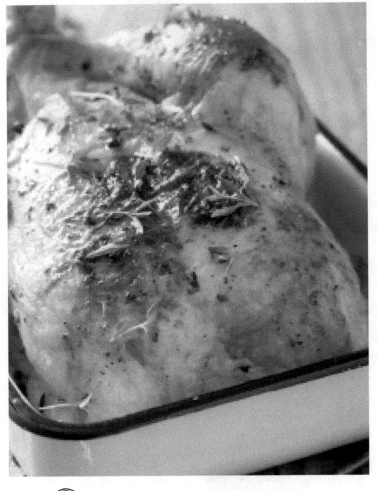

INGREDIENTS

o 2 pounds whole chicken

o 1 teaspoon of lemon zest, slivered

o 1 cup of oil-cured black olives, pitted

o 4 cloves garlic

o 1 bunch of fresh thyme, leaves picked

DIRECTIONS

1. Begin by preheating your oven to 360 degrees F. Then, spritz the sides and bottom of a baking dish with nonstick cooking oil.

2. Sprinkle the chicken with paprika, lemon zest, salt, and black pepper. Bake for 60 minutes.

3. Scatter black olives, garlic, and thyme around the chicken and bake an additional 10 to 13 minutes; a meat thermometer should read 180 degrees F.

PREPARATION
10 MIN

COOKING
60 MIN

SERVES FOR
4 PEOPLE

NUTRITION: calories 174, fat 16, fiber 3, carbs 9, protein 5

Baked Lamb with Spinach

INGREDIENTS

- o 2 tablespoons of coconut oil
- o 2-pound lamb necks, trimmed and cut into 2-inch pieces crosswise
- o Salt, to taste
- o 2 medium onions, chopped
- o 3 tablespoons of fresh ginger, minced
- o 4 garlic cloves, minced
- o 2 tablespoons of ground coriander
- o 1 tablespoon of ground cumin
- o 1 teaspoon of ground turmeric
- o 1/4 cup of coconut milk
- o 1/2 cup of tomatoes, chopped
- o 2 cups of boiling water
- o 30-ounce frozen spinach, thawed and squeezed
- o 11/2 tablespoons of garam masala
- o 1 tablespoon of fresh lemon juice
- o Freshly ground black pepper, to taste

DIRECTIONS

1. Preheat the oven to 300 degrees F.
2. In a substantial Dutch oven, melt coconut oil on medium-high heat.
3. Add lamb necks and sprinkle with salt.
4. Stir fry approximately 4-5 minutes or till browned completely.
5. Transfer the lamb right into a plate and lower the heat to medium.
6. In the same pan, add onion and sauté for about 10 minutes.
7. Add ginger, garlic and spices and sauté for around 1 minute.
8. Add coconut milk and tomatoes and cook for approximately 3-4 minutes.
9. With an immersion blender, blend the mixture till smooth.
10. Add lamb, boiling water and salt, and convey to some boil.
11. Cover the pan and transfer it into the oven.
12. Stir in spinach and garam masala and cook for about 3-5 minutes.
13. Stir in fresh lemon juice, salt, and black pepper and take off from the heat.
14. Serve hot.

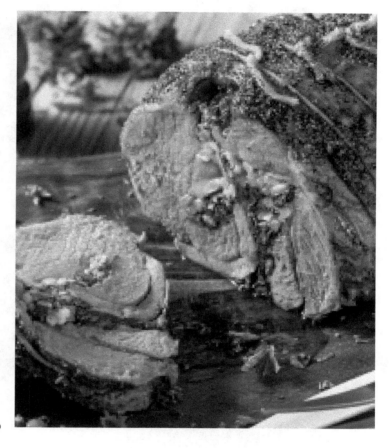

PREPARATION
10 MIN

COOKING
40 MIN

SERVES FOR
4 PEOPLE

NUTRITION: calories 424, fat 16, fiber 6, carbs 25, protein 33

Ground Lamb with Harissa

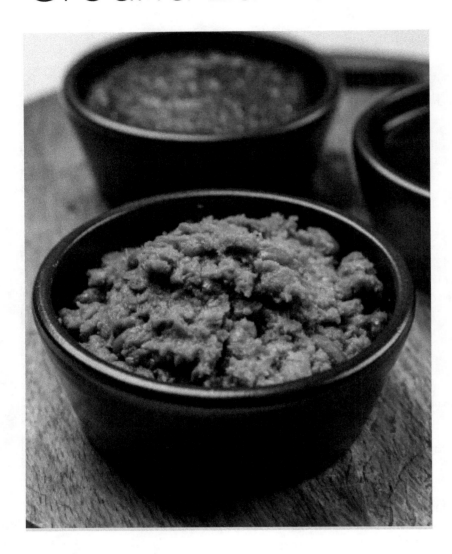

INGREDIENTS

o 1 tablespoon of extra-virgin olive oil

o 2 red peppers, seeded and chopped finely

o 1 yellow onion, chopped finely

o 2 garlic cloves, chopped finely

o 1 teaspoon of ground cumin

o 1/2 teaspoon of ground turmeric

o 1/4 teaspoon of ground cinnamon

o 1/4 teaspoon of ground ginger

o 11/2 pound of lean ground lamb

o Salt, to taste

o 1 (141/2-ounce) can diced tomatoes

o 2 tablespoons of harissa

o 1 cup of water

o Chopped fresh cilantro, for garnishing

DIRECTIONS

1. In a sizable pan, heat oil on medium-high heat.

2. Add bell pepper, onion and garlic and sauté for around 5 minutes.

3. Add spices and sauté for around 1 minute.

4. Add lamb and salt and cook approximately 5 minutes, getting into pieces.

5. Stir in tomatoes, harissa and water and provide with a boil.

6. Reduce the warmth to low and simmer, covered for about 1 hour.

7. Serve hot while using garnishing of harissa.

PREPARATION
10 MIN

COOKING
40 MIN

SERVES FOR
4 PEOPLE

NUTRITION: calories 444, fat 12, fiber 3, carbs 23, protein 37

Pork with Bell Pepper

INGREDIENTS

o 1 tablespoon of fresh ginger, chopped finely

o 4 garlic cloves, chopped finely

o 1 cup of fresh cilantro, chopped and divided

o 1/4 cup of plus 1 tbsp olive oil, divided

o 1-pound tender pork, trimmed, sliced thinly

o 2 onions, sliced thinly

o 1 green bell pepper, seeded and sliced thinly

o 1 tablespoon of fresh lime juice

DIRECTIONS

1. In a substantial bowl, mix together ginger, garlic, 1/2 cup of cilantro and 1/4 cup of oil.

2. Add pork and coat with mixture generously.

3. Refrigerate to marinate approximately a couple of hours.

4. Heat a big skillet on medium-high heat.

5. Add pork mixture and stir fry for approximately 4-5 minutes.

6. Transfer the pork right into a bowl.

7. In the same skillet, heat remaining oil on medium heat.

8. Add onion and sauté for approximately 3 minutes.

9. Stir in bell pepper and stir fry for about 3 minutes.

10. Stir in pork, lime juice and remaining cilantro and cook for about 2 minutes.

11. Serve hot.

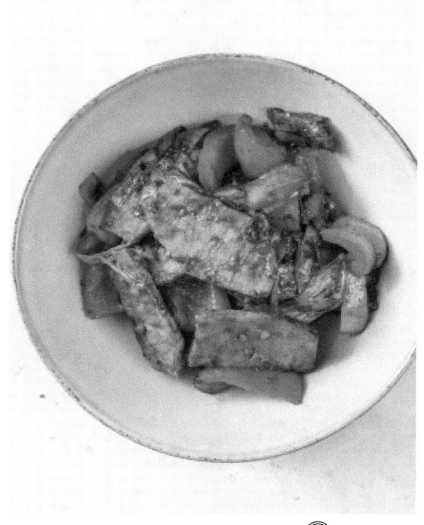

PREPARATION
10 MIN

COOKING
20 MIN

SERVES FOR
4 PEOPLE

NUTRITION: calories 429, fat 19, fiber 9, carbs 27, protein 35

Pork with Pineapple

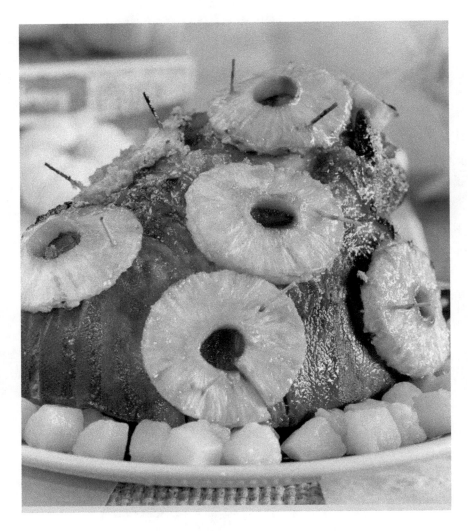

INGREDIENTS

- o 2 tablespoons of coconut oil
- o 11/2 pound of pork tenderloin, trimmed and cut into bite-sized pieces
- o 1 onion, chopped
- o 2 minced garlic cloves
- o 1 (1-inch) piece of fresh ginger, minced
- o 20-ounce of pineapple, cut into chunks
- o 1 large red bell pepper, seeded and chopped
- o 1/4 cup of fresh pineapple juice
- o 1/4 cup of coconut aminos
- o Salt and freshly ground black pepper, to taste

DIRECTIONS

1. In a substantial skillet, melt coconut oil on high heat.
2. Add pork and stir fry approximately 4-5 minutes.
3. Transfer the pork right into a bowl.
4. In the same skillet, heat the remaining oil on medium heat.
5. Add onion, garlic and ginger and sauté for around 2 minutes.
6. Stir in pineapple and bell pepper and stir fry for around 3 minutes.
7. Stir in pork, pineapple juice and coconut aminos and cook for around 3-4 minutes.
8. Serve hot.

PREPARATION
10 MIN

COOKING
15 MIN

SERVES FOR
4 PEOPLE

NUTRITION: calories 374, fat 16, fiber 3, carbs 9, protein 33

Spiced Pork

INGREDIENTS

- o 1 (2-inch) piece fresh ginger, chopped
- o 5-10 garlic cloves, chopped
- o 1 teaspoon of ground cumin
- o 1/2 teaspoon of ground turmeric
- o 1 tablespoon of hot paprika
- o 1 tablespoon of red pepper flakes
- o Salt, to taste
- o 2 tablespoons of cider vinegar
- o 2-pounds of pork shoulder, trimmed and cubed into 11/2-inch size
- o 2 cups of domestic hot water, divided
- o 1 (1-inch wide) ball tamarind pulp
- o 1/4 cup of olive oil
- o 1 teaspoon of black mustard seeds, crushed
- o 4 green cardamoms
- o 5 whole cloves
- o 1 (3-inch) cinnamon stick
- o 1 cup of onion, chopped finely
- o 1 large red bell pepper, seeded and chopped

DIRECTIONS

1. In a food processor, add ginger, garlic, cumin, turmeric, paprika, red pepper flakes, salt, and cider vinegar and pulse till smooth.
2. Transfer the amalgamation into a large bowl.
3. Add pork and coat with mixture generously.
4. Keep aside, covered for around an hour at room temperature.
5. In a bowl, add 1 cup of warm water and tamarind and make aside till water becomes cool.
6. With the hands, crush the tamarind to extract the pulp.
7. Add remaining cup of hot water and mix till well combined.
8. Through a fine sieve, strain the tamarind juice inside a bowl.
9. In a sizable skillet, heat oil on medium-high heat.
10. Add mustard seeds, green cardamoms, cloves, and cinnamon stick and sauté for about 4 minutes.
11. Add onion and sauté for approximately 5 minutes.
12. Add pork and stir fry for approximately 6 minutes.
13. Stir in tamarind juice and convey with a boil.
14. Reduce the heat to medium-low and simmer for 11/2 hours.
15. Stir in bell pepper and cook for about 7 minutes.

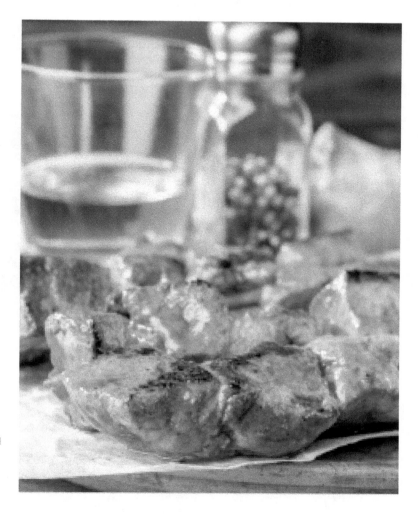

PREPARATION
10 MIN

COOKING
50 MIN

SERVES FOR
4 PEOPLE

NUTRITION: calories 435, fat 16, fiber 3, carbs 9, protein 40

Tenderloin Steaks with Caramelized Onions

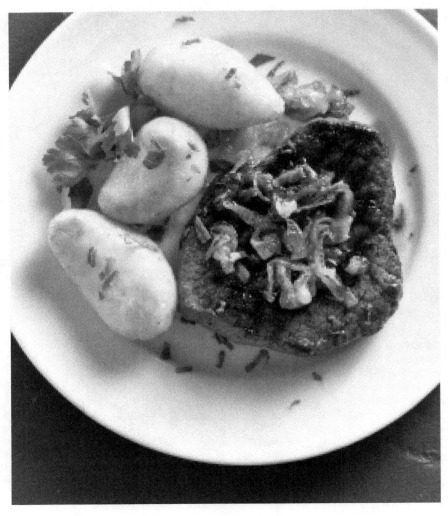

INGREDIENTS

o 4 pcs of 4-oz beef tenderloin steaks, trimmed

o 1/4 tsp ground black pepper

o 1 tsp dried thyme

o 1/2 tsp salt, divided

o 2 tbsp honey

o 2 tbsp red wine vinegar

o 1 large red onion, sliced into rings and separated

DIRECTIONS

1. On medium-high fire, place a large nonstick fry pan and grease with cooking spray.

2. Add onion, cover, and cook for three minutes.

3. Add 1/4 tsp salt, honey, and vinegar. Stir to mix and reduce fire to medium-low.

4. Simmer until sauce has thickened around 8 minutes. Stir constantly. Turn off fire.

5. In an oven-safe pan, grease with cooking spray add beef. Season with pepper, thyme, and remaining salt.

6. Pop into a preheated oven on high and bake for 4 minutes. Remove from oven and turnover tenderloin pieces. Return to oven and bake for another 4 minutes or until desired doneness is achieved.

7. Transfer to a serving plate and pour onion sauce over.

Serve and enjoy.

PREPARATION
10 MIN

COOKING
20 MIN

SERVES FOR
4 PEOPLE

NUTRITION: calories 174, fat 16, fiber 3, carbs 9, protein 5

Lamb Burger on Arugula

INGREDIENTS

- 2 tbsp shelled and salted Pistachio nuts
- 1/2 oz fresh mint, divided
- 1 tbsp salt
- 3 oz dried apricots, diced
- 2 lbs. ground lamb
- 4 cups of arugula

DIRECTIONS

1. In a bowl, with your hands blend salt, 1/2 of fresh mint (diced), apricots, and ground lamb.

2. Then form into balls or patties with an ice cream scooper. Press ball in between a palm of hands to flatten to half an inch. Do the same for the remaining patties.

3. In a nonstick thick pan on medium fire, place patties without oil and cook for 3 minutes per side or until lightly browned. Flip over once and cook the other side.

4. Meanwhile, arrange 1 cup of arugula per plate. Total of 4 plates.

5. Divide evenly and place cooked patties on top of arugula.

6. In a food processor, process until finely chopped the remaining mint leaves and nuts.

7. Sprinkle on top of patties, serve and enjoy

PREPARATION
10 MIN

COOKING
6 MIN

SERVES FOR
6 PEOPLE

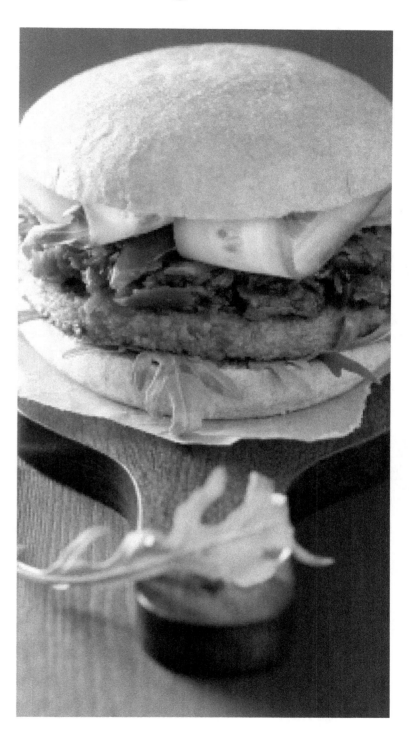

NUTRITION: calories 332, fat 20, fiber 1, carbs 6, protein 32

Cashew Beef Stir Fry

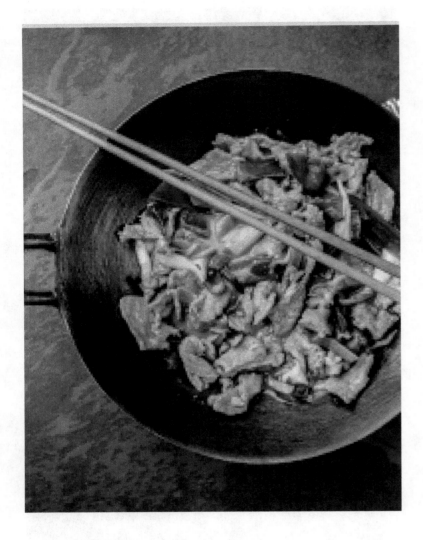

INGREDIENTS

o Salt and pepper to taste

o 1 small can water chestnut, sliced

o 1 small onion, sliced

o 1 red bell pepper, julienned

o 1 green bell pepper, julienned

o 1/4 cup of coconut aminos

o 1 tablespoon of garlic, minced

o 2 tablespoons of ginger, grated

o 1 1/2 pound ground beef

o 2 teaspoon of coconut oil

o 1 cup of raw cashews

DIRECTIONS

1. Heat a skillet over medium heat then add raw cashews. Toast for a couple of minutes or until slightly brown. Set aside.

2. In the same skillet, add the coconut oil and sauté the ground beef for 5 minutes or until brown.

3. Add the garlic, ginger, and season with coconut aminos. Stir for one minute before adding the onions, bell peppers and water chestnuts. Cook until the vegetables are almost soft.

4. Season with salt and pepper to taste.

5. Add the toasted cashews last.

PREPARATION
10 MIN

COOKING
15 MIN

SERVES FOR
8 PEOPLE

NUTRITION: calories 332, fat 20, fiber 1, carbs 6, protein 32

Beefy Cabbage Bowls

INGREDIENTS

- 1/2 teaspoon of paprika
- 2 cups of beef broth
- 1 cup of cauliflower rice
- 1 garlic clove, minced
- 1 medium head cabbage, cored and chopped
- 1 tablespoon of dried marjoram
- 1-pound lean ground beef
- 2 tablespoons of raisins
- 8-ounces tomato sauce
- 1 tbsp oil
- Salt and pepper to taste

DIRECTIONS

1. Place a heavy-bottomed pot on medium high fire and heat pot for 2 minutes.

2. Add oil and heat for 2 minutes.

3. Add the beef. Season with salt and pepper. Cook the beef until it is browned. Add the garlic and marjoram. Cook for a few minutes.

4. Add the tomato sauce, beef broth, paprika, and raisins.

5. Bring to a boil and boil for 5 minutes. Lower fire to a simmer and simmer until beef is fork-tender, around 60 minutes.

6. Adjust seasoning. Stir in rice and cabbage and boil for 5 minutes.

7. Turn off the fire and let it rest for 10 minutes.

Serve and enjoy.

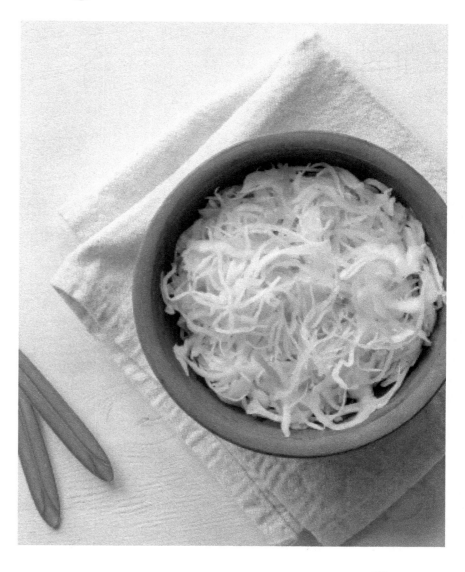

PREPARATION
10 MIN

COOKING
80 MIN

SERVES FOR
4 PEOPLE

NUTRITION: calories 342, fat 17, fiber 4, carbs 16, protein 34

Chapter 14: Desserts Recipes

Finikia

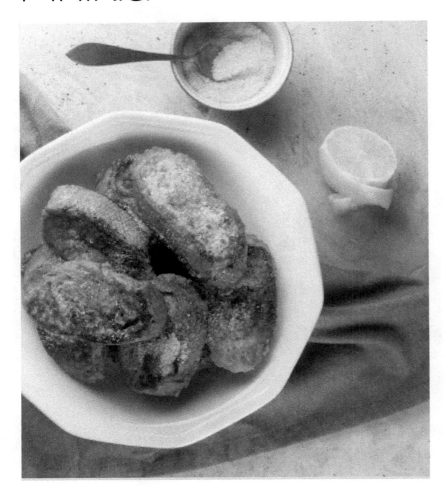

INGREDIENTS

- o 1/2 teaspoon lemon zest, grated
- o 4 tablespoons of Erythritol
- o 4 tablespoons of semolina
- o 2 tablespoons of olive oil
- o 8 tablespoons of wheat flour, whole grain
- o 1 teaspoon of vanilla extract
- o 1/2 teaspoon of ground clove
- o 3 tablespoons of coconut oil
- o 1/4 teaspoon baking powder
- o 1/4 cup of water

DIRECTIONS

1. Make the dough: in the mixing bowl combine lemon zest, semolina, olive oil, wheat flour, vanilla extract, ground clove, coconut oil, and baking powder.

2. Knead the soft dough.

3. Make the small cookies in the shape of walnuts and press them gently with the help of the fork.

4. Line the baking tray with the baking paper.

5. Place the cookies in the tray and bake them for 20 minutes at 375F.

6. Meanwhile, bring the water to boil.

7. Add Erythritol and simmer the liquid for 2 minutes over the medium heat. Cool it.

8. Pour the cooled sweet water over the hot baked cookies and leave them for 10 minutes.

9. When the cookies soak all liquid, transfer them to the serving plates.

PREPARATION
15 MIN

COOKING
20 MIN

SERVES FOR
6 PEOPLE

NUTRITION: calories 165, fat 11.7, fiber 0.6, carbs 23.7, protein 2

Vasilopita

INGREDIENTS

o 1 egg

o 3 tablespoons of butter, softened

o 1 teaspoon of baking powder

o 1/3 cup of Erythritol

o 1 teaspoon of vanilla extract

o 1/2 cup of almond meal

o 1/2 cup of wheat flour, whole grain

o 1 teaspoon of orange zest, grated

o 1/4 cup of milk

o 1 tablespoon almond flakes

DIRECTIONS:

1. Mix up together butter and Erythritol and start to mix it with the help of the cooking machine for 4 minutes over the medium speed.

2. Meanwhile, crack the egg and separate it into the egg yolk and egg white.

3. Add egg yolk in the butter mixture and keep mixing it for 2 minutes more,

4. After this, whisk the egg white till the strong peaks.

5. Add egg white to the butter mixture.

6. Then add vanilla extract and orange zest.

7. When the mixture is homogenous, switch off the cooking machine.

8. Add almond meal, wheat meal, and milk.

9. Mix up the dough until smooth and transfer it to the non-sticky round cake mold.

10. Flatten the surface of the cake with the help of the spatula and sprinkle with almond flakes.

11. Bake vasilopita for 40 minutes at 345F.

12. Chill the cooked pie well and cut on the.

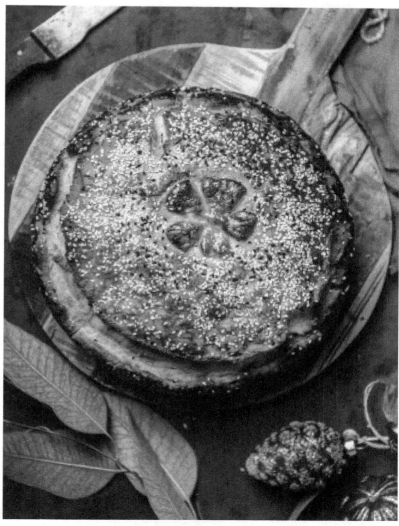

PREPARATION
20 MIN

COOKING
40 MIN

SERVES FOR
4 PEOPLE

NUTRITION: calories 245, fat 17.4, fiber 2.3, carbs 36.4, protein 6.6

Vanilla Biscuits

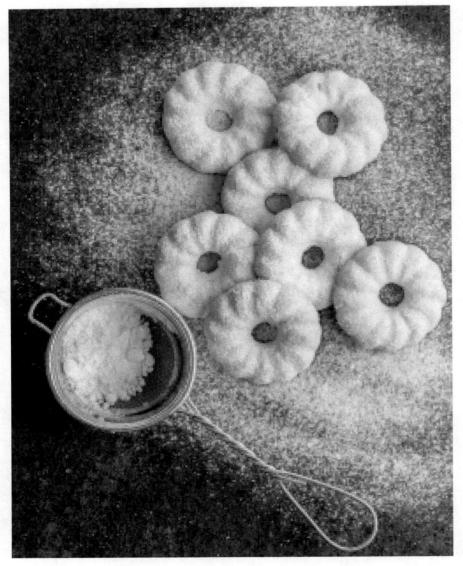

INGREDIENTS

- o 5 eggs
- o 1/2 cup of coconut flour
- o 1/2 cup of wheat flour
- o 1/3 cup of Erythritol
- o 1 teaspoon of vanilla extract
- o Cooking spray

DIRECTIONS

1. Crack the eggs in the mixing bowl and mix it up with the help of the hand mixer.

2. Then add Erythritol and keep mixing the egg mixture until it will be changed into the lemon color.

3. Then add wheat flour, coconut flour, and vanilla extract.

4. Mix it up for 30 seconds more.

5. Spray the baking tray with cooking spray.

6. Pour the biscuit mixture into the tray and flatten it.

7. Bake it for 40 minutes at 350F.

8. When the biscuit is cooked, cut it on the serving squares.

PREPARATION
15 MIN

COOKING
40 MIN

SERVES FOR
6 PEOPLE

NUTRITION: calories 132, fat 4.7, fiber 4.3, carbs 28.3, protein 7

Blueberry Cream Cones

INGREDIENTS

o 4 oz cream cheese

o 1-1/2 cup of whipped topping

o 1-1/4 cup of fresh or frozen blueberries

o 1/4 cup of blueberry jam or preserves

o 6 small ice cream cones

DIRECTIONS

1. Start by softening the cream cheese then beat it in a mixer until fluffy.

2. Fold in jam and fruits.

3. Divide the mixture into the ice cream cones.

Serve fresh

PREPARATION
10 MIN

COOKING
0 MIN

SERVES FOR
6 PEOPLE

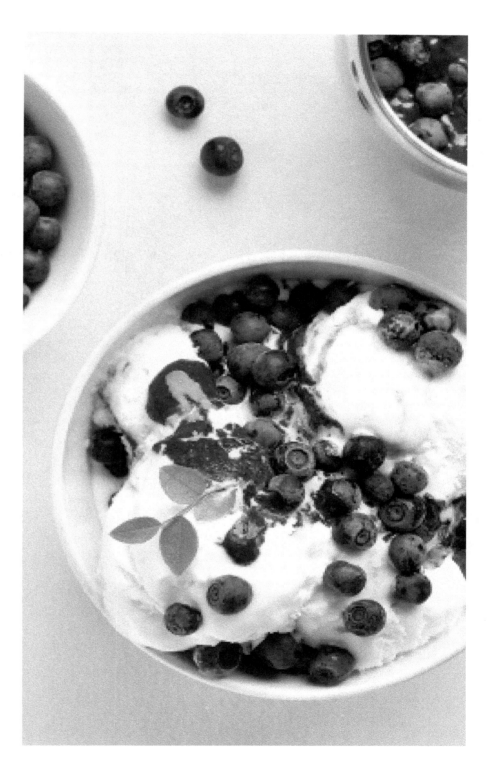

NUTRITION: calories 332, fat 20, fiber 1, carbs 6, protein 32

Cherry Coffee Cake

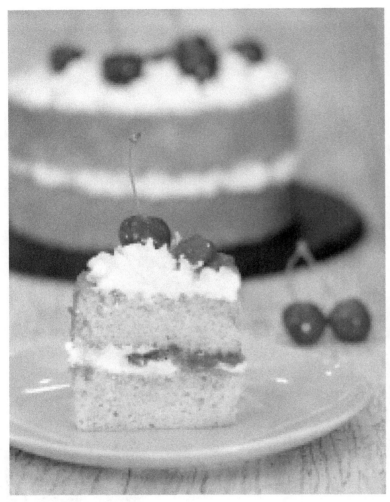

INGREDIENTS

- o 1/2 cup of unsalted butter
- o 2 eggs
- o 1 cup of granulated sugar
- o 1 cup of sour cream
- o 1 tsp vanilla
- o 2 cups of all-purpose white flour
- o 1 tsp baking powder
- o 1 tsp baking soda
- o 20 oz cherry pie filling

DIRECTIONS

1. Preheat oven to 350 degrees F.

2. Soften the butter first then beat it with the eggs, sugar, vanilla, and sour cream in a mixer.

3. Separately mix flour with baking soda and baking powder.

4. Add this mixture to the egg mixture and mix well until smooth.

5. Spread this batter evenly in a 9x13 inch baking pan.

6. Bake the pie for 40 minutes in the oven until golden on the surface.

7. Slice and serve with cherry pie filling on top.

PREPARATION
10 MIN

COOKING
40 MIN

SERVES FOR
6 PEOPLE

NUTRITION: calories 332, fat 20, fiber 1, carbs 6, protein 32

Cherry Dessert

INGREDIENTS

- o 1 small package sugar-free cherry gelatin
- o 1 pie crust, 9-inch size
- o 8 oz light cream cheese
- o 12 oz whipped topping
- o 20 oz cherry pie filling

DIRECTIONS

1. Prepare the cherry gelatin as per the given instructions on the packet.

2. Pour the mixture into an 8x8 inch pan and refrigerate until set.

3. Soften the cream cheese at room temperature.

4. Place the 9-inch pie crust in a pie pan and bake it until golden brown.

5. Vigorously, beat the cream cheese in a mixer until fluffy and fold in whipped topping.

6. Dice the gelatin into cubes and add them to the cream cheese mixture.

7. Mix gently then add this mixture to the baking pie shell.

8. Top the cream cheese filling with cherry pie filling.

9. Refrigerate for 3 hours then slice to serve

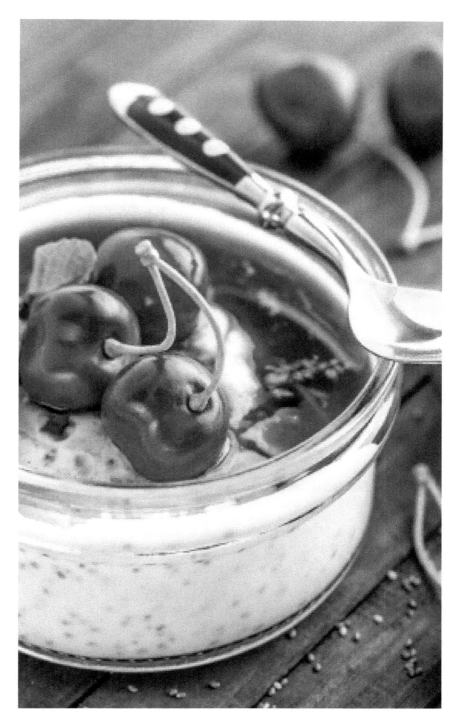

NUTRITION: calories 252, fat 20, fiber 1, carbs 6, protein 5

Crunchy Peppermint Cookies

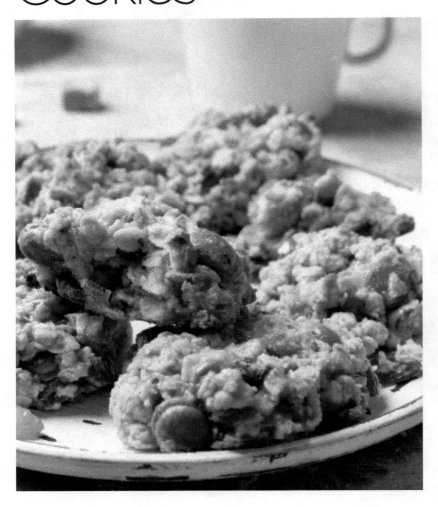

INGREDIENTS

o 1/2 cup of unsalted butter

o 18 peppermint candies

o 3/4 cup of sugar

o 1 large egg

o 1/4 tsp peppermint extract

o 1-1/2 cups of all-purpose flour

o 1 tsp baking powder

DIRECTIONS

1. Soften the butter at room temperature.

2. Add 12 peppermint candies to a Ziploc bag and crush them using a mallet.

3. Beat butter with egg, sugar, and peppermint extract in a mixer until fluffy.

4. Stir in baking powder and flour and mix well until smooth.

5. Stir in crushed peppermint candies and refrigerate the dough for 1 hour.

6. Meanwhile, layer a baking sheet with parchment paper.

7. Preheat the oven to 350 degrees F.

8. Crush the remaining candies and keep them aside.

9. Make 3/4-inch balls out of the dough and place them on the baking sheet.

10. Sprinkle the crushed candies over the balls.

11. Bake them for 12 minutes until slightly browned.

Serve fresh and enjoy.

PREPARATION
10 MIN

COOKING
12 MIN

SERVES FOR
6 PEOPLE

NUTRITION: calories 152, fat 20, fiber 1, carbs 6, protein 2

Cool Mango Mousse

INGREDIENTS

o 2 cups coconut cream, chipped

o 6 teaspoons honey

o 2 mangoes, chopped

DIRECTIONS

1. Blend together honey and mango.

2. When the mixture is smooth, combine it with whipped cream and stir carefully.

3. Put the mango-cream mixture in the serving glasses and refrigerate for 30 minutes.

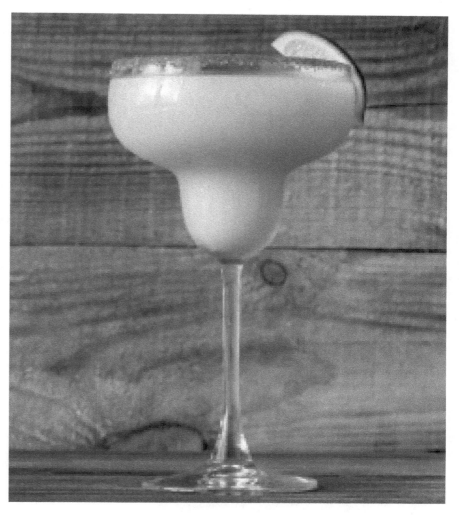

PREPARATION
8 MIN

COOKING
30 MIN

SERVES FOR
6 PEOPLE

NUTRITION: calories 272, fat 19.5, fiber 3.6, carbs 27, protein 2.8

Sweet Potato Brownies

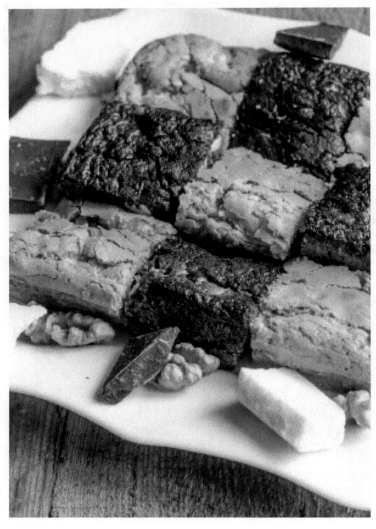

INGREDIENTS

o 1 tablespoon of cocoa powder

o 1 sweet potato, peeled, boiled

o 1/2 cup of wheat flour

o 1 teaspoon of baking powder

o 1 tablespoon of butter

o 1 tablespoon of olive oil

o 2 tablespoons of Erythritol

DIRECTIONS

1. In the mixing bowl combine together all ingredients.

2. Mix them well until you get a smooth batter.

3. After this, pour the brownie batter in the brownie mold and flatten it.

4. Bake it for 30 minutes at 365F.

5. After this, cut the brownies into the serving bars.

PREPARATION
5 MIN

COOKING
30 MIN

SERVES FOR
6 PEOPLE

NUTRITION: calories 95, fat 4.5, fiber 1.2, carbs 17.8, protein 1.6

Pumpkin Cookies

INGREDIENTS

o   1 egg, beaten

o   1 teaspoon of vanilla extract

o   1/2 teaspoon of ground cinnamon

o   1 teaspoon of ground turmeric

o   1 tablespoon of butter, softened

o   1 cup of wheat flour

o   1 teaspoon of baking powder

o   4 tablespoons of pumpkin puree

o   1 tablespoon of Erythritol

DIRECTIONS

1.   Put all ingredients in the mixing bowl and knead the soft and non-sticky dough.

2.   After this, line the baking tray with baking paper.

3.   Make 6 balls from the dough and press them gently with the help of the spoon.

4.   Arrange the dough balls in the tray.

5.   Bake the cookies for 30 minutes at 355F.

6.   Chill the cooked cookies well and store them in the glass jar.

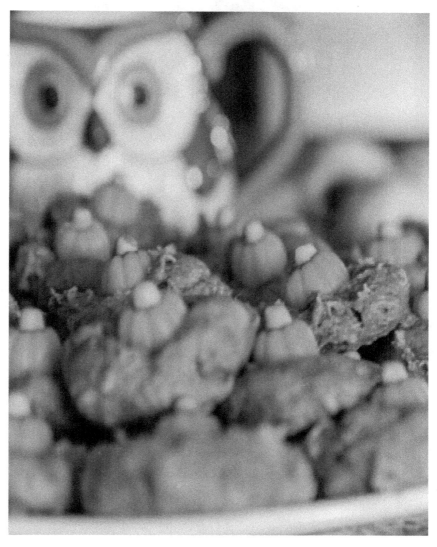

PREPARATION
10 MIN

COOKING
30 MIN

SERVES FOR
6 PEOPLE

NUTRITION: calories 111, fat 2.9, fiber 1.1, carbs 20.2, protein 3.2

Baked Plums

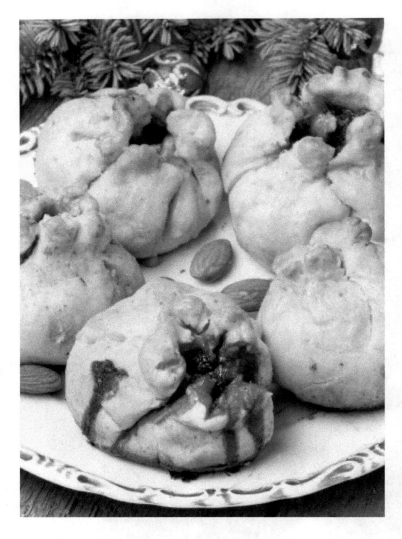

INGREDIENTS

o 4 plums, pitted, halved, not soft

o 1 tablespoon of peanuts, chopped

o 1 tablespoon of honey

o 1/2 teaspoon of lemon juice

o 1 teaspoon of coconut oil

DIRECTIONS

1. Make the packet from the foil and place the plum halves in it.

2. Then sprinkle the plums with honey, lemon juice, coconut oil, and peanuts.

3. Bake the plums for 20 minutes at 350F.

PREPARATION
8 MIN

COOKING
20 MIN

SERVES FOR
4 PEOPLE

NUTRITION: calories 69, fat 2.5, fiber 1.1, carbs 12.7, protein1.1

Classic Parfait

INGREDIENTS

o 1 cup of Plain yogurt

o 1 tablespoon of coconut flakes

o 1 tablespoon of liquid honey

o 4 teaspoons of peanuts, chopped

o 1 cup of blackberries

o 1 tablespoon of pomegranate seeds

DIRECTIONS

1. Mix up together plain yogurt and coconut flakes.

2. Put the mixture in the freezer.

3. Meanwhile, combine liquid honey and blackberries.

4. Place 1/2 part of the blackberry mixture in the serving glasses.

5. Then add 1/4 part of the cooled yogurt mixture.

6. Sprinkle the yogurt mixture with all peanuts and cover with 1/2 part of the remaining yogurt mixture.

7. Then add the remaining blackberries and top the dessert with yogurt.

8. Garnish the parfait with pomegranate seeds and cool in the fridge for 20 minutes.

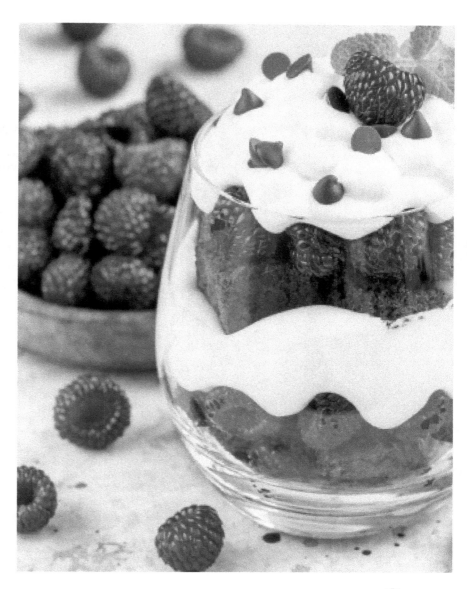

PREPARATION
10 MIN

COOKING
20 MIN

SERVES FOR
4 PEOPLE

NUTRITION: calories 115, fat 3.1, fiber 3, carbs 13, protein 5.1

Melon Popsicles

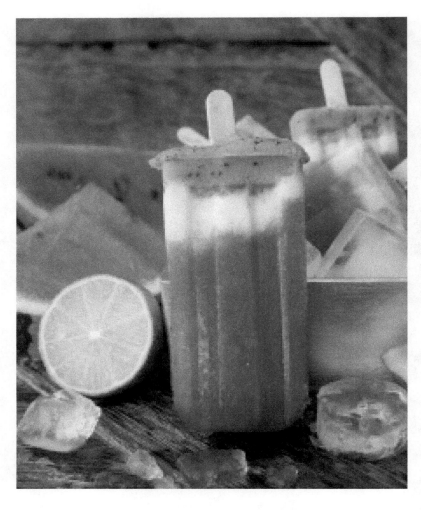

INGREDIENTS

- o 9 oz melon, peeled, chopped
- o 1 tablespoon of Erythritol
- o 1/2 cup of orange juice

DIRECTIONS

1. Blend the melon until smooth and combine it with Erythritol and orange juice.

2. Mix up the liquid until Erythritol is dissolved.

3. Then pour the liquid into the Popsicle molds.

4. Freeze the popsicles for 2 hours in the freezer.

PREPARATION
10 MIN

COOKING
10 MIN

SERVES FOR
4 PEOPLE

NUTRITION: calories 332, fat 20, fiber 1, carbs 6, protein 32

Chapter 15: Measurements and Conversion tables

VOLUME EQUIVALENTS (LIQUID)

US STANDARD	US STANDARD (OUNCES)	METRIC
2 tablespoons	1 fl. oz.	30 mL
1/4 cup	2 fl. oz.	60 mL
1/2 cup	4 fl. oz.	120 mL
1 cup	8 fl. oz.	240mL
11/2 cups	12 fl. oz.	355 mL
2 cups or 1 pint	16 fl. oz.	475 mL
4 cups or 1 quart	32 fl. oz.	1 L
1 gallon	128 fl. oz.	4 L

OVEN TEMPERATURES

FAHRENHEIT (°F)	CELSIUS (°C) APPROXIMATE
250 °F	120 °C
300 °F	150 °C
325 °F	165 °C
350 °F	180 °C
375 °F	190 °C
400 °F	200 °C
425 °F	220 °C
450 °F	230 °C

VOLUME EQUIVALENTS (LIQUID)

US STANDARD	METRIC (APPROXIMATE)
1/8 teaspoon	0.5 mL
1/4 teaspoon	1 mL
1/2 teaspoon	2 mL
2/3 teaspoon	4 mL
1 teaspoon	5 mL
1 tablespoon	15 mL
1/4 cup	59 mL
1/3 cup	79 mL
1/2 cup	118 mL
2/3 cup	156 mL
3/4 cup	177 mL
1 cup	235 mL
2 cups or 1 pint	475 mL
3 cups	700 mL
4 cups or 1 quart	1 L
1/2 gallon	2L
1 gallon	4 L

WEIGHT EQUIVALENTS

US STANDARD	METRIC (APPROXIMATE)
1/2 ounce	15 g
1 ounce	30 g
2 ounces	60 g
4 ounces	115 g
8 ounces	225 g
12 ounces	340 g
16 ounces or 1 pound	455 g

Conclusion

Even with a disease that limits so many foods, you can still make delicious treats and meals with the alternatives provided. You can also customize them according to your palate so that the food you eat not only helps your body but also boosts your mood. You can share these tasty renal-friendly meals with your friends and family and live a long life with them by your side!

There are a lot of different ways to maintain your health and to ensure that you sustain it for longer. The number one reason why patients are urged to stay healthy during the early stages of kidney disease is to avoid dialysis for as long as possible.

This can be done by incorporating the right types of nutrients in your diet, all of which are included in the right amount, in the renal diet. Maintaining your activity levels, getting enough sleep, and quitting bad habits, such as smoking and alcohol, will support your journey towards staying healthy and avoiding dialysis.

Even though there is no cure for chronic kidney disease, it is a journey that you can manage. You can sustain your health and continue living your life as normal, with a high quality of life, for much longer than if you don't follow these basic guidelines.

The number one thing to remember on this journey is that you are in complete control of your outcome.

Thank you

9 781914 164194